MOM FORGOT MY BIRTHDAY

A DAUGHTER'S JOURNEY THROUGH ALZHEIMER'S

SONYA JURY

Kansas City, Missouri

Cover design: J. Robert "Bob" Farley II, whereforeartdesign.com

Cover photo: Sonya Jury

Cover illustration copyright © Sonya Jury. All rights reserved.

Editor & Guiding Light: Lisa Allen, poet + essayist

Editing: Amy Sinnott

Interior layout: Ben Wolf, Inc.

ISBN: 979-8-218-32792-7 (softcover)

ISBN: 979-8-9897995-0-3 (ebook)

First Printing, 2024

Printed in The United States of America

CONTENTS

For my Mom, Willa Dean,
I love you gobs and gobs.

This is a journey that in a million years, I did not expect to take. This is my story and I hope it enlightens you and your family and prepares you for end-of-life care. Never did I think Alzheimer's or dementia would be part of my life or my mother's. Then, **BAM!** There it is, a big old Mack truck hitting me hard.

I write this book to share my journey, which I hope will better prepare others to be caregivers or advocates. It's not a "how-to-guide," but rather a diary of a journey of discovery that I took with my Mom starting in May 2012 and ending in April 2017. I am grateful her journey did not drag on for years. While those words might seem harsh, the reality of the cruel disease is harsher.

I do not wish Alzheimer's disease on anyone, and we desperately need a cure; fast! The statistics for Alzheimer's disease are overwhelmingly off the charts. In 2022, more than 6 million Americans of all ages had Alzheimer's. An estimated 6.5 million Americans aged sixty-five years and older are living with Alzheimer's. About 1 in 9 aged sixty-five years and older (10.7 %) has Alzheimer's. To those who have been or are currently on the caregiver journey, may peace and patience find you. May your guilt cease. I hope you find comfort and the confidence that you are doing the right thing and making the right choices because this is your journey, and you know your loved one's wishes.

What is dementia? What is Alzheimer's? As you will read, from the beginning, the doctors diagnosed her with dementia, using it as an umbrella term. I would later learn that Alzheimer's nests itself within dementia and there are many forms and stages. Dementia means it is severe enough to interfere with daily life, which was my Mom's case. She started with mild cognitive impairment which escalated into dementia in a few short months. Alzheimer's is a brain disease that destroys memory and thinking skills. In my Mom's case, the doctor asked her to draw a circle representing the face of a clock, place the numbers on the clock's face, and then draw the hands of the clock to a specific time. When Mom drew the clock face, all of her numbers were squished to one side of the circle clock face—definite dementia diagnosis. All this knowledge I discovered on this journey. I didn't just wake up one day and have all the answers. It was all trial and error. And err I did.

The Alzheimer's Association's website is filled with knowledge related to both dementia and Alzheimer's. As I began writing this book, I found a perfect explanation from www.alz.org[1] website which succinctly describes the stages:

Early-stage Alzheimer's (mild)

In the early stage of Alzheimer's, a person may function independently. He or she may still drive, work, and be part of social activities. Despite this, the person may feel as if he or she is having memory lapses, such as forgetting familiar words or the location of everyday objects.

Symptoms may not be widely apparent at this stage, but family and close friends may take notice and a doctor would be able to identify symptoms using certain diagnostic tools.

Common difficulties include:

- Coming up with the right word or name
- Remembering names when introduced to new people
- Having difficulty performing tasks in social or work settings
- Forgetting material that was just read
- Losing or misplacing a valuable object
- Experiencing increased trouble with planning or organizing

Middle-stage Alzheimer's (moderate)

Middle-stage Alzheimer's is typically the longest stage and can last for many years. As the disease progresses, the person with Alzheimer's will require a greater level of care.

During the middle stage of Alzheimer's, the dementia symptoms are more pronounced. The person may confuse words, get frustrated or angry, and act in unexpected ways, such as refusing to bathe. Damage to nerve cells in the brain can also make it difficult for the person to express thoughts and perform routine tasks without assistance.

Symptoms, which vary from person to person, may include:

- Being forgetful of events or personal history
- Feeling moody or withdrawn, especially in socially or mentally challenging situations

- Being unable to recall information about themselves like their address or telephone number, and the high school or college they attended
- Experiencing confusion about where they are or what day it is
- Requiring help choosing proper clothing for the season or the occasion
- Having trouble controlling their bladder and bowels
- Experiencing changes in sleep patterns, such as sleeping during the day and becoming restless at night
- Showing an increased tendency to wander and become lost
- Demonstrating personality and behavioral changes, including suspiciousness and delusions or compulsive, repetitive behavior like handwringing or tissue shredding.

In the middle stage, the person living with Alzheimer's can still participate in daily activities with assistance. It's important to find out what the person can still do or find ways to simplify tasks. As the need for more intensive care increases, caregivers may want to consider respite care or an adult day center so they can have a temporary break from caregiving, while the person living with Alzheimer's continues to receive care in a safe environment.

Late-stage Alzheimer's (severe)

In the final stage of the disease, dementia symptoms are severe. Individuals lose the ability to respond to their environment, carry on a conversation, and, eventually, control movement. They may still say words or phrases, but communicating pain becomes difficult. As memory and cognitive skills continue to worsen, significant personality changes may take place and individuals need extensive care.

At this stage, individuals may:

- Require round-the-clock assistance with daily personal care
- Lose awareness of recent experiences as well as of their surroundings
- Experience changes in physical abilities, including walking, sitting, and, eventually, swallowing
- Have difficulty communicating
- Become vulnerable to infections, especially pneumonia

The person living with Alzheimer's may not be able to initiate engagement as much during the late stage, but he or she can still benefit from interaction in appropriate ways like listening to relaxing music or receiving reassurance through gentle touch. During this stage, caregivers may want to use support services, such as hospice care, which focuses on providing comfort and dignity at the end of life. Hospice can be of great benefit to people in the final stages of Alzheimer's and other dementias, as well as their families.

After reading the above, it hit me that this was my Mom's journey precisely. As you read this book, you will move through my nonlinear memories to the best of my recollection. These stories and memories became pieces of a larger puzzle as I worked to understand and solve the many challenges during Mom's illness. It is meant to be raw, brutally honest, and very uncomfortable at times. It is my story of pure, naked vulnerability at its best. It is not meant for you to pity me or the experience we lived through. At times, I felt I was in a reality TV show and some of these experiences...you couldn't make up. Life does happen. If any part of my experience helps you, then I will take comfort in that.

Peace,
　Sonya

PART 1

EARLY-STAGE ALZHEIMER'S (MILD)

MAY 2012 – MAY 2015

SOMETHING'S NOT RIGHT
MAY 2012

Wednesday

I arrived home from work that night in May around 8:00 p.m. When my cell phone rang, it was Mom.

Me: *"Hi, Mom. How are you?"*
Walt: *"Hi, Sonya. It's Walter."*

> **Walt never calls me.**
> **This can't be good.**

Me: *"Hey, Walt. How are you?"*
Walt: *"I'm fine, but your Mom isn't, and I don't know what to do."*
Me: *"What's wrong?"*
Walt: *"She has diarrhea really bad, she's on the toilet, and I can't get her to move. She's just not herself."*
Me: *"Ok, um, can you put her on the phone?"*
Walt: *"I'll try…"*

In the background, I hear them talking.

Walt: *"Dean, Sonya wants to talk to you."*
Mom: *"No, I'm fine. Why did you call her?"*
Walt: *"Please, Dean. Talk to her."*
Mom: *"OK."*–as he hands her the phone.
Me: *"Hi, Mom. How are you? What's going on?"*
Mom: *"Sonya, I've got diarrhea so bad. Dr. Punkie told me to take Imodium and I have been, but it just won't stop."* (Coughing spell) *"I'm fine, just leave me alone."*
Me: *"Mom, if you don't feel good, let Walt take you to the hospital to get checked out."*
Mom: *"Hell, no. I don't need to go to the hospital. I don't know what you and he are all worried about. I'll be fine."*
Me: *"Mom, put Walt back on the line."*
Walt: *"Hello?"*
Me: *"I'm hopping in the car, and I'll be there in about forty minutes. I'll go with you to take her to the ER in Harrisonville."*
Walt: *"Thank you."*

I quickly change into comfy clothes, not knowing how long of a night I have ahead of me at the ER. I quickly feed and walk our dog Tucker, as my husband Scott was out of town. I hop into my orange VW Beetle and speed toward Pleasant Hill, Missouri. Of course, my mind is racing. Mom sounded agitated and confused, even combative. What happened? For months she had complained about diarrhea, but this time something else was wrong. It had to be.

Right?

I pull into the farm, park the car, and walk to the front door. (Past all the flowers and weeds in the front flower bed.) When Mom and her second husband Walt retired, they wanted to be in the country. They purchased a *circa* 1970, 3,000-square-foot ranch home on twenty acres of land, with three bedrooms, three full baths, a family room, a dining room, and a kitchen. The house also had a full basement with another kitchen, family room, and bedrooms. The property had the typical country red barn with a gabled roof, a red 50' x 100' metal barn, and another red 10' x 10' wooden garden shed. They loved this place and were proud to call it home. Over the last couple of years, the flower beds became too much for Mom and the weeds took over. Walt continued to plant his large garden with tomato plants, cucumbers, peppers, and jalapenos. Now that I think about it, that had even become too much for them.

Once inside the house, I witnessed the concern on Walt's face. Dean is never sick and now he is taking care of her. He knows this isn't right and the fear or confusion shows.

I hugged Walt and headed toward the hall bathroom.

Now, I realize that finding your Mom sitting on the toilet is not the image any of us want. But picture that and hold that thought. I peek around the door frame.

Me: *"Hi, Mom. What's going on?"*
Mom: *"Sonya, I don't understand it. Dr. Punkie kept telling me to take Imodium and it would all be better. I've been taking Imodium the last four months, and it isn't getting any better."*

I can tell something isn't right. Her voice is shaky, she is confused, combative, and cursing up a storm. Not my Mom. She is coughing and trying to clear her throat constantly. She takes her index finger and presses it against the back of her throat to clear something. I turn to look at Walt. With a knowing glance, we both understand that we need to take her to the ER.

Over the next fifteen minutes, I begged and pleaded with Mom to let us take her to the hospital. Reluctantly, she gave in.

I work to calm her and get her off the toilet. Once we help her get dressed, we tell her we are going to take her to the hospital to figure out what is wrong and why her diarrhea won't go away.

Me: *"Mom, can you make the car ride to the hospital?"*
Mom: *"Yes, I can make it."*

Walt grabs her purse and verifies that her ID and insurance cards are there. We fuss around a bit to ensure all is well, diarrhea-wise, before beginning the thirty-minute drive to the Cass Regional Medical Center ER in Harrisonville. We help her to the car and get her buckled in. I say I will follow them to the hospital. I hug and kiss her. I tell her everything will be fine. Off we go.

Here I am, driving down the dark country road, headed to the local hospital to check my Mom into the ER.

> *What's up with sticking her finger in*
> *her mouth/down her throat? What is*
> *that going to achieve?*

All these rational questions and emotions are hitting all at once.

> *Rational, that's a word that will*
> *haunt me over the next five years.*

Memory is a funny thing. As I am driving, my mind starts flickering through images of a happy, healthy Mom. I am transported back to 1977, when Mom, dad, my brother Bob, and I lived in a different ranch home at the end of a cul-de-sac, surrounded on two sides by soybean fields on the outskirts of Columbus, Ohio. Mom and dad always had an affinity for living in the country. I guess it gave them comfort from their upbringing in Kentucky. Now, here I was driving down a dark country road, following Walt and Mom in their burgundy, four-door Lincoln Town Car. I have this vivid memory of Mom driving us through the dark Ohio country-side, in a two-door, dark-green International Scout for the thirty-minute, once-a-week trip to Delaware, Ohio. Dad was always traveling, and Mom and I would make it an event. We would dine at the local Burger Chef. Mom would special order a fish sandwich for me, no cheese or tartar sauce. A special order meant we would need to wait for the cook to prepare it. Mom would order her usual cheeseburger. On the AM radio, we would listen to the local country western station, and if lucky, Elvis, the Statler Brothers, or Dolly Parton would come on. We would listen intently while making small talk about what I had learned at school that day.

The three of us arrive at the hospital and escort her into the ER. Of course, the small rural hospital has a wait! I shake my head. While waiting, she continues to cough and put her finger in her mouth. She also begins asking the same questions repeatedly.

Me: *"Mom, please stop putting your finger in your mouth."*

Mmm, this is a new behavior.

While waiting, we make small talk. She is agitated and doesn't like us doting on her.

Me: *"Mom, stop putting your finger in your mouth."*

I notice the distrust building in her facial expressions. She looks at me with…what is that look? Disdain? Curiosity? I have not seen this before. She is not her cheerful Mom self.

Once in the ER, the doctor orders the typical work-up.

Cheerful Mom is all about pleasing others. You want a batch of chocolate chip cookies; chocolate cookies are on their way. You want a French Silk pie; she will make you one. You need your pants hemmed; not a problem. Mom would greet anyone with a smile and never met a stranger. She loved being around people, listening to their stories, and sharing hers. She was a true joy.

And now we wait in the ER hospital room engaging in small talk.

The tests came back, and they highlighted that her sodium level had dropped. The doctors believe it is due to the diarrhea and dehydration. The nurse starts an IV to rehydrate, and the medical staff believes she will be fine by morning. She is admitted and they will contact her primary care doctor, Dr. Punkie, to swing by and check her out tomorrow. Once settled into her room, Walt and I say our goodbyes and head home. It's a bit after midnight. We walk to the parking lot chatting about Mom and her recent change of behaviors.

Walt shares that she has become more forgetful and a bit aggressive when she does forget something. He shares that she has become paranoid with everyone, including him. I ask for examples. He references her cooking, saying she recently burned a blackberry cobbler.

Mom burned a cobbler?

This lady, who loves to cook, does not burn cobblers, especially sweets!

This is not normal.

We say our goodbyes and head to our respective homes. I tell Walt I'll be back first thing in the morning to ensure I am there when the doctor stops by on rounds.

Thursday

The next day, I arrive at the hospital by 7:00 a.m. Mom is sleeping soundly, which means she is snoring like a banshee! I chuckle and smile. Walt is also asleep in a chair next to her. He later shared that once he got home, Mom called crying, scared, and begging him to come back to the hospital. He did. While this might not seem unusual, for my Mom it was. It was a red flag I did not understand.

Her behavior had definitely changed; suddenly, she was needy. She was not the independent, happy-go-lucky Mom we all knew.

Dr. Vincent, Dr. Punkie's medical partner, arrived midmorning to examine her and take vitals. They would be running a few more tests, including a repeat of the sodium level test. The doctor ordered a CT scan and told us she had lacerated her uvula. When she put her index finger in her mouth, she was doing it to "clear her throat" to stop the coughing, but what she was actually doing was poking her uvula, which resulted in an enlarged uvula, perpetuating the coughing. Once we realized this action, we continually told her to stop putting her finger in her mouth. All of this led to a combative discussion fueled by paranoia.

I suggested Walt go home, take a nap, a shower, and come back later. I would hang out with Mom during the day. I had my laptop and would work from her bedside. While Walt was away, Mom launched into long ramblings about Walt, his kids, and life insurance policies. She was upset that Walt had not updated his life insurance policy and that Walt's "no-good kids" would inherit money. You see, Mom was not a fan of Walt's two adult children, Lynn and Sandy. Daughter Sandy had floated in and out of rehab, lost her job with the government, and hopped from job to job to make ends meet. Sandy only called Walt when she needed something—money.

Walt's son Lynn and his family lived in Salt Lake City, and once a year they would make the obligatory family visit to see Mom and Walt. Mom tolerated the visit because she knew it would make Walt happy. Mom would always find a way to call me during Lynn's visit to vent; of course, I listened.

Friday

Her sodium level has returned to within the normal range, but Mom has not returned to *her* normal self. The doctors are a bit puzzled that she has not bounced back fully. They want to keep her overnight, run a few more tests to dig a little deeper, and rule out other diagnoses. She continues to show aggressive tendencies with a bit of paranoia. Her dialogue turns to rants about money, life insurance policies, how Walt is keeping things from her, and Walt's children. It's not normal for her.

Mom loves Walt more than any human could. Her behavior has changed. Now she was belittling him, she was being completely disrespectful, and showing him no compassion or love. She was not Cheerful Mom.

Saturday

There was no change in her behavior and still a bit of diarrhea. With plenty of time on my hands, I decided it would be a good chore to empty her purse and clean it out. Like any good Mom at the age of seventy-four, her purse was filled with tissues, papers, mints, pennies, two tubes of lipstick, toothpicks, Chapstick, and a wallet. What I didn't expect to find were all the used and unused wrappers of Imodium tablets.

> ***This is odd. Lightbulb! Had she been
> popping these pills like candy?***

Here was another red flag I didn't clue in on at first—her memory. She didn't remember taking a pill, so she popped another one.

Sunday: Mother's Day

I was back at Cass Regional Medical Center early so I would not miss the doctors' rounds. Dr. Vincent came in around noon. Mom was calmly sitting in bed with a bit of a dazed, skeptical look toward him. Here it comes, the explanation of what is wrong with Mom. Dr. Vincent matter-of-factly says Mom has dementia.

> ***Dementia. I will need to Google that later.***

Dr. Vincent shares that dementia can be a catch-all for illnesses when another terminology or diagnosis doesn't quite fit. While Alzheimer's could be the actual diagnosis, I knew enough to know that one cannot confirm Alzheimer's until a person has passed and an autopsy is performed on their brain. At this point, I hadn't conducted my research on dementia or Alzheimer's and didn't know what was in our future. Dr. Vincent stated that Mom would need full-time care to ensure she took her medication on time. Her short-term memory was failing and soon so would her long-term memory. It was also apparent she was not going to be the cook, or the cleaner, or be able to do any of the other household duties she gladly accepted. In a matter of days, Walt went from being taken care of by Mom to being catapulted into the caregiver role. Walt didn't know what that meant, but he loved her and would do what it took. Dr. Vincent gave

Walt the book *The 36-Hour Day* by Mace and Rabins to read. In hindsight, I should have read it as well.

They released Mom from the hospital on Mother's Day 2012. Bewildered, we all left together. Walt took Mom home. My husband Scott and I went to Walmart to fill her prescriptions, pick up a few groceries, and order dinner from Mazzio's Pizza to take to the farm.

Considering all we had been through over the last several days, dinner was refreshingly typical with stories and laughter. Mom was still agitated and wanted to recap her experience. She was highly frustrated with all the doctors and her victim mentality was out in full force. She declared she would no longer see Dr. Punkie, who had been her primary care physician for a couple of years. Adamantly, she proclaimed that Dr. Vincent would be her new primary care doctor. It did help that Dr. Vincent and Dr. Punkie were in the same practice. She was livid that Dr. Punkie kept telling her to take the Imodium and everything would be fine; that didn't make sense to me either. Walt was tired and you could see it in his eyes. He was not a guy to share emotions. Rather he would hold them close, and they would weigh on him. We finished dinner, and Scott and Walt cleaned up everything. I led Mom back to their bedroom to get dressed and ready for bed. She continued to repeat questions, and I did my best to be supportive and reassuring. All the while, internal angst and anxiety brewed inside me.

Me: *"Good night, Mom. I love you."*
Mom: *"Good night, Sonya. Thank you for taking care of me. I love you, gobs and gobs."*

Over the next several days, I called to check in on Mom and Walt. Even though I am a Type A personality, and I so wanted to jump in and take control, I respected their privacy and knew they needed time to work through their new normal. In the meantime, I read everything I could about Alzheimer's, dementia, and caregivers to arm myself with knowledge.

We were all exhausted and hopeful that normalcy would return for all. I was not prepared mentally, emotionally, or physically for the journey ahead. Scott and I drove back home to Kansas City. It was an incredibly quiet car ride home.

As I laid my head upon my pillow...

***Goodnight, Mom. I truly hope you sleep well
and overcome whatever this is.***

Mom's Voicemail: 20 May 2012, at 10:14 a.m.

"Uhm, Good Morning, Sonya. It's...it's Mom. Honey, I am calling to apologize for how our conversation ended last...yesterday afternoon. I am so sorry for any of the things I said that hurt your feelings in any way. Please...just bear with me and everything. If you talked with Walt, you will see what a magnificent recovery that I have met...made. And I am not going back to Punkie anymore. I don't know if Dr. Vincent will be able to take me or not. But then, I may go back to the doctor that I had at Overland Park. So anyway, I just want to call and apologize. I, I, I tell you, I have no madness whatsoever towards you or...um...Scott. I love you kids with all of my heart. So, that's what...wa...had to say, to let you know this morning. I love you all and thank you for all you have done. Bye-bye."

2

A SECOND CHANCE

MAY 1987

It was a little after 10:00 p.m. when I pulled into my parents' driveway. I was returning home after the two-hour drive from Manhattan, Kansas, having had dinner with my boyfriend Scott Jury. He was graduating from Kansas State University, and I was not able to attend his graduation due to a European trip that had been planned for a year. My classmate and I were leaving in two days to fly to Chicago to obtain a new passport (thanks to the French Consulate losing my original passport) and then a visa from the French Consulate. From there we would fly to Amsterdam, catch an overnight bus to Paris, and meet our other friend, Steve Smith, under the Arc de Triomphe on Monday at 10:00 a.m. All these arrangements were made via letters and phone calls; cell phones and the internet did not exist yet. Three architecture geeks were headed to Europe to see all the buildings we had studied in architectural history class. I was giddy to begin our European travels.

I had made my "Sonya Lasagna" for Scott to celebrate his graduation and say our goodbyes. After graduation, Scott would head to Europe too. First to Greece and maybe, just maybe, he would find me in Spannochia, Italy, where I was to study architecture for the summer.

Pulling into the driveway, I immediately noticed dad's yellow Mercury Grand Marquis was not there. That was odd; I knew he wasn't traveling.

Where was dad?

I gathered my things and walked into a noticeably quiet house. Mom was seated on the loveseat, wearing her pink JC Penney nightgown and robe. She was waiting for me. The house was eerily silent, and I knew she was the only one in the house. Her husband, my dad, John Likins, was not there. A calm of lightness washed over me as I looked into her eyes. I immediately felt a burden lifted.

What was her face telling me?

Me: *"Hi, Mom. Where's dad? What's going on?"*
Mom: *"Hi, Sonya. Sit down, I need to tell you something."*

Over the next hour, she confided in me everything she had held back for the last ten years since moving to Kansas City. She shared she no longer loved dad, and his constant infidelity was too much to bear. His recent job loss and selling of tools, guns, and other belongings was not acceptable. He had cashed out all the International Harvester bonds they had tucked away for a rainy day. He had drained their bank account and set up his own. She realized he was liquidating everything they, and she, had worked toward. She had confronted him, and he finally gave her the answer she needed to hear: "I don't love you." That was enough for her to make the decision she had fretted over. Even as a small child, I remember thinking to myself, Mom and dad do not love each other.

Mom: *"Sonya, I filed for divorce and the sheriff served the papers here at the house and escorted him away. We don't need him anymore. It's just the two of us."*

My heart broke for her. At the same time, I was thrilled that she finally stood up for herself. We hugged and cried. I was completely dumbfounded, elated, and proud of her. This moment was the turning point in our lives where we both were free to be who we wanted, say what we wanted, laugh when we wanted, and live how we wanted without the constant looming fear of him. What's the saying? Don't poke the bear?

This life event gave me a newfound love, respect, and friendship with Mom. She was brave. This was her shining moment, and whatever I could do to ensure her happiness, I would do it. I was so immensely proud of her. I wanted her to experience unending happiness and joy—as much as the world could offer. She deserved it after all those years of living unhappily in a loveless marriage.

3

MY BIRTHDAY

MAY 2012

A few weeks after Mom's dementia diagnosis, my forty-seventh birthday fell on Memorial Day, May 28. I like to think I gave everyone in the United States the day off to celebrate. I called Mom every few days since her stint at the hospital earlier in the month to check in and see how she and Walt were doing. I wanted to hear her voice and see if there had been a change with her. When we spoke, she sounded like Normal Mom. Maybe a bit forgetful, but really Normal Mom. For the days leading up to my birthday weekend, I would go to the mailbox with certainty and anticipation to find a birthday card stuffed in a brightly colored envelope, covered with birthday stickers, and addressed in Mom's cursive handwriting. Each day I went to the mailbox. Each day I was disappointed.

This was the first time, **EVER**, Mom forgot my birthday. Shock and bewilderment crept over me. I felt wronged!

Why would Mom forget my birthday?
How could Mom forget my birthday?
What was going on with her?

I remember having a conversation with Scott about her forgetting my birthday. I was harsh, unempathetic, and miffed even. She loved making birthdays special for everyone. She loved celebrating you on your special day. As a kid, she would always bake us homemade cakes with the sweet Duncan Hines box of frosting. Chocolate cake was my favorite and she graciously obliged. The cake would be complete with those fat birthday numbers shoved into the top of the cake to commemorate your special year. I loved it when she baked because I always got to lick the mixing beaters clean of frosting. I have so many fond memories of all the birthday cakes she made for me over the years.

This year would be different.

No birthday cake.

No birthday card.

No "Happy Birthday!" phone call.

I never received a birthday card from her again. I knew she was different, yet I didn't understand or want to understand why or how. I could not comprehend her change.

Nor did I want to accept it.

Mom's Voicemail: 29 May 2012, at 6:10 p.m.

"Hey, congratulations, Sonya. This is Mom. This morning I opened the paper and guess whose picture I saw right there? Yours! Congratulations! I cut it out and it's in the folder with all the rest of the things. I like the orange dress you had on. So…I really like orange. So…have a good week. I love you all. Bye-bye."

4

THEIR NEW NORMAL
OR SIGNS I MISSED
SUMMER 2012

After Mom's diagnosis, I did my best to support Mom and Walt's privacy, so they could work into their new normal. When I would call Mom during the week, our conversation was very one-sided. If I asked a question, she would ask Walt for the answer; she could not remember events. The cooking was now up to Walt, which meant trips to the local Walmart for frozen foods. Sure, Mom could make simple things—cornbread, bacon, eggs—but ask her to follow a recipe and she would forget ingredients as the dementia progressed.

One random Saturday, before her diagnosis, we visited them, and Mom made lunch—chicken enchilada casserole and a French Silk pie for dessert. She was herself in the kitchen; it was her happy place. While making lunch, she stopped a couple of times in the middle of the kitchen to collect her thoughts about the next task she needed to complete. Lunch was great as always that day. A few random signs were there, but I missed them.

Over the next few months, their lives seemed to return to normal, except for a few hindsight quirks.

Mom loved her flowers and gardening. They defined her.

She would spend hours digging, planting, weeding, and watering to create the perfect flower bed. She loved it when folks visited, and she could walk them through her creations naming every single plant. Yeah, I have this trait too. Her flower vignettes were filled with love and the occasional garden statue, or a repurposed item like an old boot. An old boot was a perfect container for her favorite succulent called mother of hens. After her diagnosis, she lost all interest in flowers, the gardens shriveled up, and the weeds won out.

Looking back, she had also lost interest or confidence in driving. She always loved to drive. She learned to drive at a young age and now had no interest. Several months before, she would think nothing of hopping in her trusty maroon Rav4 and meeting me at a halfway point to spend the afternoon together in Kansas City. Now, no way. When I questioned her about it, she shrugged it off and said she just didn't want to meet me.

Was this a sign I missed?

Mom's asking for permission. As I look back, about a few years before her diagnosis, when I would ask her to do anything, she would need to clear it with Walt while I was on the phone. Walt would always say yes. It annoyed the heck out of me because she never would have asked permission before. She was a woman of action, but now she needed validation or reassurance from Walt. I often wonder if this was a signal and I missed it.

LESSON 1: Be conscious of tasks they love and now have no interest in. Watch for signs.

The last signal I missed was shiftiness, or rather, her ability to compensate with a bit of creative redirecting. I do not mean this in a derogatory way but in a crafty way. Mom knew something wasn't quite right with her. When you would have a conversation or she would forget something, she was quick to joke about it, shrug it off, and redirect your attention to something else. Something other than her.

Here is a list of behavior changes/lack of interest with Mom that I missed:

- Driving
- Gardening
- Cooking
- Asking Walt for permission
- Asking Walt to validate a comment/statement she would make
- Needing more than normal validation from Walt
- Withdrawal from social activities, such as the ladies' church luncheons
- Withdrawn during social events
- Disorganized house (normally everything had a place)
- Cluttered desk with Post-it note after Post-it note, all with the same information
- Phone calls every day when normally we would talk every week; she began to forget more
- Misplacing of items
- Forgetting she had taken her medications
- Lack of concentration and focus

Mom's Voicemail: 1 August 2012, at 5:32 p.m.

"Hi, Sonya. It's Mom. I just haven't talked with you for a week or so, so I miss talking to you, honey. Thought I'd give you a call. I

have to go to the dentist tomorrow. I am dreading it so bad because I know I have to have some...oh...extra work. Don't quite know what it's going to be in everything, the bridge that I have just don't seem to fit right anymore. So anyway I'm really dreading it but anyway. So, I'll call me when you have time. Love you all. How are you, Scott? So...will talk to you...when you give a call. Bye."

MOM LOVES WALT
1990

Mom began dating a bit after her divorce from my dad was final in 1988. Yet no one caught her eye. She had several first dates, and our roles were reversed at home. I would wait for her to return to the house after her date. I loved hearing about the guy, the dinner, and their conversation. Girl talk at an adult level.

Mom and Walt met through work at the family-run business of Farris Burns located in Merriam, Kansas. Walt was the metal shop supervisor, keeping the business humming along, and Mom worked as the bookkeeper, keeping the financials organized. Their relationship started as a working relationship until Mom's divorce from my dad.

Once Mom's divorce was final, and the same for Walt, their relationship changed, and each day they grew fonder of each other. After Walt left his not-so-happy relationship, they were free to pursue each other. They were inseparable and loved each other's company. They could sit on any given afternoon and talk about anything and everything.

They just clicked and began dating. This would include Saturdays driving around the countryside, shopping at antique stores or estate sales, and dinner out. When two people have a second chance at love, it's fun to watch how they work harder in a relationship and let the little things fade away.

If I am being honest, Walt was not my first choice for Mom. Would anyone be the right person?

Um, No

Walt made her happy, and I had to remind myself of that. Even Scott would remind me, on occasion, that Walt dearly loved "his Deanie." He was a softy at heart and quite romantic, giving her flowers and a lovely senti-mental card for each anniversary and birthday. Mom saved every anniversary card they exchanged during their twenty-year marriage in an old hat box.

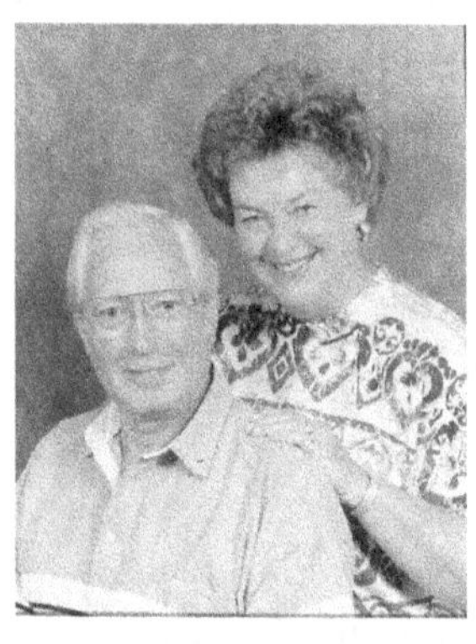

Mom loved Walt and doted on him. She loved to cook for him, so much so, in their first years together they collectively gained about thirty-five pounds! Eating made both of them happy.

Suddenly, they switched roles that May of 2012.

WALT THE CAREGIVER
OCTOBER 2012

Caregiver is a big word with so much meaning. The definition is a family member or paid helper who regularly looks after a child or a sick, elderly, or disabled person. The most common type of caregiver is a family caregiver (a.k.a. informal caregiver), which is what Walt had become overnight.

The types of caregivers:

- Professional
- Independent
- Private
- Informal
- Volunteer

Within the caregiver family, some facilities exist to provide these services:

- Adult daycare centers
- Nursing homes
- Assisted living
- Home health care
- Hospice

Each of the above categories has specific definitions, and they are constantly evolving to meet the demands of the various stages of dementia/Alzheimer's. For example, there now exists a virtual caregiver option. I am not claiming to know everything, yet only wish to provide a bit of context; it is darn confusing at times! A decoder ring would be nice.

Mix in the confusion of the various stages of the disease, the different caregiver levels, and facilities. Add a dash of your own anxiety, stress, and uncertainty about how to handle this subject. Know it is not easy. Confusion and uncertainty are normal. You will find what works for you.

Fast forward to October 2012. Scott and I were on vacation at Rosemary Beach, Florida. Mom called to inform me that she had to call 911 for Walt. He was having difficulty breathing. He was now in the Cass Regional Medical Center with a diagnosis of bacterial pneumonia. In May, after her dementia diagnosis, Walt was catapulted as her caregiver, and he wore himself out. Walt so adored Mom and he wanted to be the loving, brave husband and take care of her. He also had a stubborn streak and didn't like asking for help from others.

Taking care of a loved one with dementia is hard work—plain and simple. You will wear yourself out. I know you are reading this and thinking, "No way, I can do it." The truth is yes, you *can* do it, and it will take its toll on you as well.

Dr. Vincent gave Walt the book *The 36-Hour Day* to read. It is an excellent resource for families thrown into caring for people who have dementia-related diseases. The challenge and irony is finding the time to actually read the book. There is a reason the authors chose the title. As a full-time caregiver, you are on point for what feels like a thirty-six-hour day. Not only are you taking care of your basic needs—sleep, food, shower, medications, grocery shopping, work, safety, and life itself—you are consumed with ensuring your loved one is taking her pills in a timely manner, doesn't inadvertently hurt herself or you, eats, sleeps, and brushes her teeth. Many of you have raised a young child and remember the constant repetition of the word, "Why?" Now, you are taking care of an older adult who, before now, could take care of themselves. It messes with your mind.

Did he even have the time to read the book?

Walt decided to take care of his Deanie. As he would say, it was his marital duty—in sickness and in health. I can support his love and duty, but it killed him. He was stubborn and proud and did not want anyone to come into their home and help with the laundry, cleaning, or cooking. He wouldn't stand for it. He wasn't my dad, and I didn't have the confidence to pressure him. Hindsight is 20/20. I should have pushed harder.

As a caregiver, he took over the cooking, cleaning, laundry, church meetings, and writing notes everywhere in the house. He kept track of medications—hers and his. He was doing it all.

He truly did a yeoman's job caring for her and it wore him out. Think about that last sentence for a moment. Imagine being seventy-eight years old and taking care of an adult with cognitive impairment that manifests in childlike qualities. She began constantly asking questions and a lot of them included, "Why?" She constantly needed reassurance. She would ask the same question over and over. If an answer was not satisfactory to her, she would become agitated. Anger and paranoia would set in. When she did try to cook, Walt would sit at the kitchen table, watching from afar to ensure she didn't inadvertently burn the house down. Not only are you taking care of yourself but them too. *Exhausting* doesn't even describe the magnitude of pressure.

Lesson 2: Ask For Help and Take It! Put your oxygen mask on first.

After Scott and I returned home, I got in my VW Beetle and drove to Cass Regional to see Mom and Walt and hopefully have a conversation with Dr. Vincent who was now family doctor to both of them. Walking into the sterile hospital room that 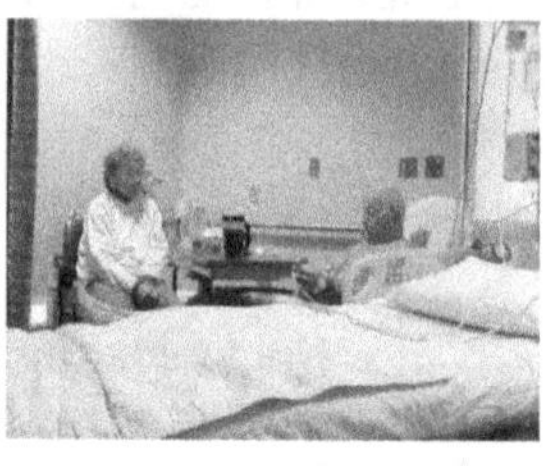 Wednesday afternoon, I had a strange feeling of unknown dread, unsureness of what was going on, or how this would affect me. I was there to support Mom if she needed it.

At this point, Dr. Vincent was somewhat optimistic that Walt would recover. Yet, if I look back, in his words he indicated to me that Walt would not recover from this, due to the type of pneumonia he had, the complications of his years of smoking (back in the day), COPD, and yearly bouts of bronchitis. Now I have a Mom with dementia and a stepfather in the hospital with pneumonia, and I was thrown into instant caregiver mode. I don't type this to gain your admiration or empathy. This was life in all its ickiness, staring us down.

Lesson 3: Ask the medical staff to speak to you in clear terminology. Just say it, even if it is hard to say and hear.

For the next ten days, Mom lived at our house in Kansas City, thirty-minutes away from Walt's hospital room. Those ten days of me being the full-time caregiver were very hard. Yes, Scott helped and supported both of us. Yet by parental proxy, I felt the weight on me. I was not my best. I did not have patience for her. I was pissed that their stubbornness of not getting all of their affairs in order was landing on us to deal with. More on this later.

My new routine: wake-up, get dressed, do a bit of work, fix something to eat, organize Mom, and take her to the hospital to keep Walt company. Mom was still self-sufficient in that she could dress and feed herself. Her dementia challenges at this point were her memory, and not having the ability to make a rational decision, or understand what was happening. In her mind, Walt would heal, and they would return to the farm. Pneumonia had another plan.

Walt was moved from rural Cass Regional Medical Center to the main urban hospital, Research Medical Center, thirty-minutes away, on a Friday afternoon. The doctors said it was in his best interest, and heading into the weekend, Walt needed to be in an ICU that could handle his pending issues. This should have been an even bigger red flag for me, but I missed it. What the doctors were saying but not saying–Walt would need a ventilator, and the local hospital did not want to deal with it. They needed the mothership hospital to take on his case.

When we arrived at Research Medical Center, the nurses got him settled into ICU. While this was happening, a doctor pulled me aside to have *the conversation*. Walt had a severe case of bacterial pneumonia and if his oxygen level dipped to a certain point, a ventilator was imminent. Again, I missed the clues. The doctor asked if Walt had a living will, DNR, or power of attorney. None that I was aware of.

> *In my head, I am thinking, shit! I knew*
> *this was going to happen. Scott and I*
> *had been asking, begging, for them*
> *to get their affairs in order.*

Shit, shit, shit

I shared with the medical staff that Mom, due to her dementia, was not capable of making a rational life decision. I knew enough about Mom's mental state, and she would want everything to be done to save her Walter. This is, of course, a rational human decision. Yet the doctors were subtly trying to inform us of what was happening. Walt was not my father; I was not his daughter and, therefore, did not have the authority to make this life-or-death decision.

The nurses were empathetically supportive of Mom and Walt. They had witnessed this movie on many occasions. As I watched the doctors and nurses buzz around both Mom and Walt, you could see the movie playing out in the staff's heads. If you were intentionally looking, you could see it in their eyes, and the frustration of not knowing what decision would be made if Walt needed a ventilator. The doctor tried to talk to me about asking Walt to sign a life directive order. I asked Walt if he would sign a life directive. Of course, if any of us were put into that exact moment, no one would sign a life directive. Would you? Here is where I wish the doctors would have been empathetically blunt with me about Mom and Walt. My cortisol-filled lizard brain had me amped up. I was not seeing the signs or hearing the words they were trying to convey. I didn't understand the situation.

During the past few days, Scott was out of town on business. Like any good human, he knew I needed him. So that Friday afternoon, he made his first stop back in Kansas City to see me at Research Medical Center while I was babysitting Mom and Walt.

He texted that he had arrived, and I popped out of Walt's ICU room. It was the quintessential movie scene where two lost loves see each other for the first time and run toward each other to hug and kiss. (I am not making this up!) As I ran through the ICU to greet Scott, out of the corner of my eye, I spotted Mom returning from a restroom break. My eyes met Mom's as I watched her eyes roll back, her body twirled around, and she dropped to the floor and hit her head on a column as she fell.

Are you kidding me? WTH!?

Simultaneously, Scott and I ran to Mom's aid. Thank goodness we were in the ICU, and the nurses swarmed to help. She was placed on a gurney and transported to the emergency room in the same damn building!

Yes, now both adults were in the same hospital, just in different departments. Scott and I checked in with Walt to tell him what had just happened and that we would be back to report on Mom. It must have been so hard for Walt to lay in the ICU bed, knowing his wife was being wheeled to the ER for God knows what was wrong with her. Yet in my mind, my concern was only about Mom.

Off to the ER, we went!

Mom had fainted and it was determined Mom's sodium level had dropped again. A few years back, after a visit to her dentist, Mom began having severe facial pain in her right side. The doctor diagnosed it as trigeminal neuralgia (TN). It involves sudden, severe facial pain, which can happen in an instant. To control her pain she took daily medication. After running tests, the new doctor (not her family doctor) wanted to stop that medication and start her on another one.

Lesson 4: Ask lots of questions!

I didn't ask the all-important questions:

- Should she stop her medication cold turkey OR do we wean her off it?
- Does this medication work with her current medications?
- What are the side effects of stopping all at once?
- Will her trigeminal neuralgia pain come back immediately?
- What question should I be asking that I am not?
- Any concerns?

The doctor wanted to admit her for overnight observation, which meant if she was admitted on a Friday night, she would not be released until Sunday. Selfishly, I was fine with this, as it gave me a reprieve from care-

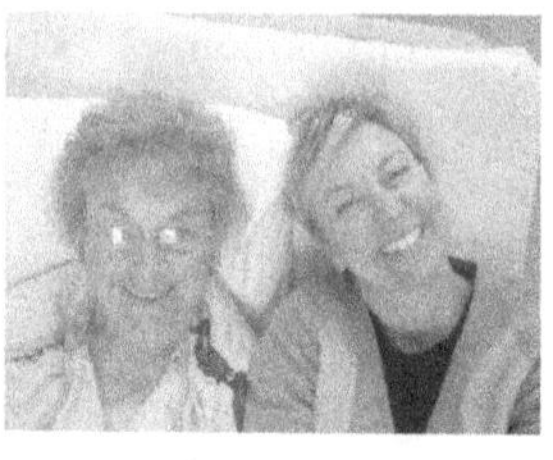

giving for a few days. Scott and I had a couple of date nights that equated to driving to the farm to look for any important legal papers that might exist.

Mom was settled in for the night in her hospital. We popped down to the ICU to let Walt know what was going on and say our good nights with him. As I left the ICU room, Walt said to me, *"Don't be so hard on me."*

It was all I could do to not lose my shit.

I bit my tongue, smiled, looked him in the eyes, and said good night.

Me: *"Good night, Walt. I will see you in the morning."*

Those were the only words I could utter at the time because I was trying to be supportive, yet inside me a tornado of emotions were swirling around. I was mad. I felt trapped. I was sad for both Mom and Walt, for me, for all of us. I was frustrated with the entire scenario. I genuinely thought I was living in my own reality TV show. The plot was thickening...

Here, lying in an ICU bed, was a scared man who knew he would eventually die. He knew it, and I knew it. By both of their inactions, they were now imposing life decisions on their children (my brother Bob; Walt's children, Lynn and Sandy; and me) because they were too darn stubborn and naïve to create a living will and power of attorney or share their life-or-death decisions with anyone!

LESSON 5: Share your life-or-death decisions with everyone!

We left the hospital and went to the nearest bar for drinks and food.

Drink we did. We vented, laughed, and cried. I am so incredibly grateful for Scott. He listened and supported me through this experience unconditionally. He learned when to listen and when to offer an opinion or support. He learned to love me more selflessly than any human could. To this day, I am eternally blessed with an incredible life partner.

The next day, Scott and I drove to the farm to search for any and all important legal papers, if any existed. We brought back five boxes filled with information we would need to sift through. Our evenings over the next several months consisted of us making dinner, sitting outside by the fire pit with a wine glass in hand, and reading through every single piece of paper. We had to look at every piece of paper because they both had developed an unbelievably bad habit of writing their Social Security numbers on everything! If it wasn't important, or if it was over seven years old, I pitched it into the fire pit. Wine and fire—very cathartic.

Burn, baby, burn.

7

MY ROCK

May each of you have someone in your life who is your pillar you can lean on during your journey. You will need one or several. I was fortunate to have mine—Scott.

My husband, J. Scott Jury, was born in Wichita, Kansas, to Ann and Jack Jury. Scott is the youngest of three kids, his sister Cathy, who is seven years older, and his middle brother Cliff. Scott and I met on New Year's Eve, December 31, 1986, in a Kansas City bar called Confetti's. It was love at first sight for me. I'm not sure what it was about him. Maybe it was his infectious smile, kind and caring eyes, wicked sense of humor, dance moves, intelligent conversation, or the whole package. He is a good man, and I am grateful for his love. Scott asked me to marry him on March 10, 1990, and we settled on a Kansas City wedding date of September 29, 1990. The wedding was simple; we were surrounded by friends and family. We were two young kids in love, not understanding or knowing what a marriage was all about. We learn from our parents what goes into a marriage. My parents divorced while I was in college, and I knew I did not want my marriage to be like theirs. My parents showed me what *not* to do.

Scott's parents had a solid marriage, a true partnership filled with love. Scott and I both leaned toward this definition of marriage.

My brother Bob, his wife Faith, and their two wickedly smart daughters made the drive from Wilmington, Ohio to attend our wedding. Bob walked me down the aisle on the big day and he was there for the "father of the bride" dance too. With Walt on her arm, Mom beamed the entire wedding day; weddings were her jam. She loved being the center of attention as the mother of the bride. She loved a good celebration! It was a good wedding day.

The cliche of two people learning to live together is true. You learn to lean on each other and your lives ebb and flow with the rhythm of career, life, friends, and family. I am extremely grateful we lived in Indianapolis for the first five years of our marriage. We could build our foundation without the interference of family. To this day, I look back on those years with nostalgic fondness. It shaped us for whatever life threw at us. Neither one of us knew, yet, what it means to lose a Mom to lung cancer, a father to glioblastoma, dear friends to heart attacks, or a Mom to dementia. At twenty-five years old, we were only looking ahead to Friday cocktail hour. I would like to think all our experiences prepared us for dealing with Mom's dementia diagnosis, but they didn't. We took one day at a time and did our best.

Scott was my rock, and he quickly learned how best to support me. Yes, there were times when all I wanted to do was bitch about Mom's situation. Why had this happened to her? In my judgmental mind, of course, it happened to her! She did nothing to take care of herself. She never worked out. She had a diet of fried foods, processed foods, and sugary drinks. She was just so backward. In my darkest bitchy moments, Scott would remind me to see the goodness of my mother.

He'd say, "She loves you deeply, you know she does. She is a good person."

Those harsh truthful words would cut through me, make me feel horrible for feeling the way I did, and smack me back to reality. That reality would remind me that sometimes bad things happen to wonderful people. It still sucks.

Time to buck up buttercup and deal with it.

Mom loved Scott. Scott loved my Mom. When he walked into her room, she would be the first to pop up from the chair and rush to hug him, sometimes before hugging me. Scott has a natural grace with people, people are drawn to him. They want to talk to him and hear his stories and ideas. He makes people laugh, and he loves to jest with Mom and make her smile. I truly loved watching them interact.

When we would visit Mom and Walt at the farm, Mom would always cook something special for Scott—chicken enchiladas, French Silk pie, peanut butter cookies, lasagna, or Mom's good ol' roast beef with mashed potatoes and gravy. I am not a gravy fan, so Scott loved it when Mom made her special gravy. It's funny, when we knew we were going to be with Mom and Walt for a few days, both of us went on a diet, or ate lightly a few days prior. That way we didn't have too much guilt about overeating Mom's cooking.

The relationship between Mom and Scott was as good as it gets. She was happy I had met and married a wonderful man who loves her daughter and treats her well. Mom knew she had an amazing son-in-law who would always be there for her daughter and, if needed, her too. Scott was just that; he was Mom's rock, too.

LESSON 6: Find your rock.

8

____

RING, RING
OCTOBER 2012

It was 4:30 a.m., Saturday morning, and my cell phone rang.
It was the Research Medical Center ICU nurse.

Nurse: *"Your dad's oxygen level has dropped, and we need
to intubate him. Do we have your permission?"*
Me: *"I am not his daughter. I do not have power of attorney
to make any life decisions, and my Mom isn't capable at this
time. His son Lynn lives in Salt Lake City, and I don't know
where his daughter Sandy is these days. Do what you need
to do."*
Nurse: *"He keeps pushing us away as though he doesn't
want it."*
Me: *"Then he probably understands what you are trying to
do. Again, I do not have the power to tell you no, only his
kids can."*

I hung up, my stomach in knots. A tidal wave of emotions
fell over me: sadness, helplessness, lack of control, anger, and
the realization that Walt could die. Something inside of me
told me he was not coming out of this situation for various
health reasons. I sat in bed gathering my thoughts. The next

few moments turned into rote habits of getting dressed to head over to the Research Medical Center, to speak with a doctor and check in with Mom to see how she was doing.

Your mind and body go through the proverbial motions of brushing your teeth, getting dressed, and grabbing the essentials for what would seem like another eternity of sitting in a hospital, waiting.

Me: *"Scott, we need to go to the hospital."*

That Saturday morning, Walt went on a ventilator.
Let that sit for a moment.
Riding to Research, I prepared all my questions to ask the medical staff:

- Did he understand what was happening?
- Did he say anything?
- What does it mean to be placed on a ventilator?
- What was happening?
- How are his other vitals?
- What was going on with his lungs?
- How long would this last?
- Was he in any pain?
- What were the next steps?
- Could he recover from this?
- What should I prepare for?
- What do you need from me?

We walked through the double doors of the ICU department and headed toward Walt's room located at the end of the communal hallway. There was a nursing station and staging area for all the various medical equipment needed for the patients. All the fluorescent lights were turned down for the nighttime setting; it gave the ICU an eerie silence where you only heard the occasional footsteps of a nurse, an occasional groan, and the rhythmic beats of machines. As we turned the glass corner to peer into his room, seeing him lying in bed, sedated, eyes taped closed, with a tube down his throat, it was just sad. My heart ached for Mom and him. I was not trying to be a doom or gloom person; my sixth sense told me this was not good. The ICU nurse who called me was still on duty, and she was wonderful at explaining what was happening to Walt.

When intubated, the patient is sedated, and their body is put into a coma-like state so medical staff can insert a plastic breathing tube down the throat to pump oxygen into the lungs. Once a person is placed on a ventilator, they are given approximately fourteen days to "wait and see" how the patient recovers or any sign of progress. The doctors are watching oxygen saturation levels, respiratory breathing rate, and heart rate in hopes of improvement. Once fourteen days have passed, time is up and the loved ones—spouse, partner, parent, next of kin, siblings, or power of attorney—need to make another decision. The choices are to continue the ventilator or remove the ventilator and allow nature to take its course.

Dammit, I knew this was going to happen.

Up until this point, Mom and Walt had not contacted Walt's two kids. They had no idea that their dad had been in the hospital for the past week with a worsening case of bacterial pneumonia. With Mom in her state of being due to her recent fainting spell and fall, she couldn't make the call. It was time to call Walt's son Lynn in Salt Lake City and share the unfortunate news.

Dammit, I don't want to make this phone call. If only they had made a will and taken care of all the legal aspects, I would not be making this fucking call.

Do you know how difficult it is to make this call? Mom and Walt married in 1991, and I had visited with Walt's kids maybe three times in twenty years. We were not close. Maybe being distant made it easier, as I didn't have all the "loved one" emotions to pile on. I only had to deliver the raw clinical truth.

> ### *Who was I kidding?*
> ### *This was not going to be easy. Ugh.*

Standing in the fourth-floor hallway at Research Medical Center, I found a quiet location to make the call. The quiet location was the lobby area in front of the bank of four elevators, central within the hospital. As the phone started to ring, I began pacing in circles within the lobby area. I could hear my own heart racing, and I had no clue how I would tell him about his dad, yet I knew I had to.

Lynn: *"Hello?"*
Me: *"Hi, Lynn. This is Sonya Jury, Dean's daughter, and I have some not-so-good news to share with you. Walt has been battling pneumonia this last week and it took a turn for the worse. He was hooked up to a ventilator this morning. To my knowledge, Mom and Walt do not have a living will or power of attorney documentation. When the nurse called me at 4:30 this morning to ask what to do about putting Walt on a ventilator, I told her I could not make that decision, nor could Mom."*

As would be expected, Lynn was dumbfounded that his dad had been dealing with pneumonia for about a week and he knew nothing. He asked lots of clarifying questions, and I did my best to answer them factually without emotion. Again, Walt was not close to his children, and neither he nor Mom felt the need to inform them of the situation. Mom and

Walt thought this was going to be no big deal and Walt would heal and they would get to go back to the farm to live happily ever after. I did too a few days ago. Now I did not.

> **Me:** *"Lynn, Walt needs you. Please come to Kansas City to deal with the doctors."*

During the call with Lynn, I shared all the facts about his father, the timeline, his severe case of pneumonia, and why he was placed on the ventilator. I told him the nurse's comment about Walt trying to push them off as they were telling him what they were going to do. I also shared with Lynn that the decision to place someone on a ventilator is a personal or family decision that I could not make, not being his daughter. And Mom could not decide because she was incapable, due to her seizure. And as far as I knew, Mom and Walt did not have a will or any documents for what to do in this situation.

As difficult as it was to make the call, I felt bad for Lynn. Walt and his previous wife Eileen had two kids, Lynn and Sandy. From what Walt had shared, their family had unique dynamics and it was not the *Leave it to Beaver* family relationship we sometimes nostalgically use as a frame of reference. Their family struggled with drugs, alcohol, and, in my opinion, a lack of love. I had listened to Mom over the years complain about Sandy or Lynn calling Walt for money. It was an unfortunate situation, which I did my best to keep at a distance, but now I needed Lynn to be the caregiver for his dad. I still needed to maintain my focus on Mom.

After I hung up with Lynn, I took a moment to reflect on the dark irony of the situation that both Mom and Walt were in the same hospital, except one of them was unconscious! As I spoke with the ICU nurse, she was brutally honest with me regarding Walt's situation. I was sad and grateful for her kindness and willingness to tell me what to expect. I went upstairs to visit Mom and let her know what had happened to

Walt and that he had been placed on a ventilator earlier that morning. She struggled to comprehend what was happening to her Walt. We talked and cried. I did my best to be brave and comfort her. Another tough conversation. I told Mom that I would make the obligatory calls to all their friends— Pastor Todd, Walt's brother Hal, his cousin Arlen, and Walt's Mom. Little did I know I would become their lifeline during Walter's final journey.

Sunday afternoon, after a conversation with Mom's doctor regarding her fainting spell and new medication, Mom was released from the hospital. Once again, Scott and I escorted her downstairs to the ICU for her to see her beloved Walt. It was heart-wrenching to watch her kiss him, hold his hand, and speak to him. Here was the true love of her life, lying in an ICU bed, connected to machines keeping him alive, and there was nothing she could do. That feeling of helplessness is defeating. I shared with her that I had called Walt's son Lynn, and he would be arriving the next day.

We left Research and took Mom back to our house. She would stay with us for the next week while we waited to see if Walt would recover. It was a very tough week for all parties.

Mom continued to ask the same questions over and over:

"What happened to Walt?"
"Why was he on the machine?"
"When did this happen?"
"Why am I here with you?"
"When will he be ok?"
"When are we going back to the farm?"

That week of taking care of Mom was exhausting. Scott and I had many discussions about caregiving. Combined with the collective experiences of friends and family dealing with similar family experiences, we both agreed that full-time personal caregiving for Mom was not a permanent path we would, or could, continue. We knew we needed a caregiver's help to support Mom. I conducted my research and found a home health care company to spend nights and a few days with Mom at her home on the farm.

A few days after Mom's release from Research Hospital, the three of us drove down to the farm where Mom and Walt lived. I told Mom we were going to pick up a few things so she could continue to live with us until Walt was released. In reality, we were waiting to meet a home health night nurse I had hired to stay with Mom that night. Yes, it was a little white lie. The first of many.

We were all in the kitchen at the farm talking about Walt and his condition while stealthily waiting for the night-shift caregiver to arrive. Scott and I were trying to gauge Mom's cognitive ability; it was clear she was not fully comprehending what was going on with Walt and his prognosis, specifically due to her fainting spell a few days before.

Mom: *"Sonya, why is this happening? What is wrong with Walter? When will he come home?"*

I was seated at their round kitchen table, and Mom was standing in the middle of the kitchen talking. For a nanosecond, she went silent, stared off into the distance, then started to fall.

Scott: *"Sonya, catch her! She is falling!"*

At the same time Scott spoke, I sprang from the chair. Mom's eyes rolled back, and she twirled around falling toward the floor. I caught her before she hit the ground. She immediately started convulsing.

Not again!

Scott dialed 911 on the landline speaker phone. Kudos to the 911 operator for talking us through everything, asking questions, and calmly giving us the support we needed. Yes, it seemed like an eternity watching Mom writhe on the floor, convulsing. The paramedics were there within fifteen minutes. If you have not had the experience of paramedics descending upon your home, it is a well-orchestrated process. Scott and I stood back helplessly watching. I didn't cry. I just stood there replaying everything in my mind from the past several days. My emotions were worn slick, and I didn't have anything else to give. I felt helpless, defeated, and so sad for her, for me, for this situation. The paramedics got her hooked to an IV, loaded her in the ambulance, and off they went to take her to Lee's Summit Medical Center, a twenty-minute drive.

After everyone left, Scott and I stood in the kitchen hugging and looking at each other in unfathomable wonder.

Did this just happen?

How surreal this moment was. Only ten days prior, Scott and I were enjoying the sunshine and sand at Rosemary Beach, Florida, with amazing friends. On the flight back to Kansas City, we both were thinking that whatever was going on with Walt would be no big deal. He would be in the hospital for a few weeks and get out of this. Everyone's life would go back to normal. It was not meant to be.

Only a few days prior, during my first drive to the Cass Regional Medical Center to meet up with Mom and Walt to discover what was going on, I still didn't understand the severity of the bacterial pneumonia coursing through Walt's lungs. Even when I met with Dr. Vincent by myself (when he commented on pneumonia being an old man's grim reaper visiting), I didn't hear what he meant.

Instinctively, my action-mode skill set took over. Knowing

we were not going to be making a trip back to the farm anytime soon, we took a few extra moments to grab a few boxes with important papers. We gathered a few more of Mom's clothes and personal items. We turned on a few night lights throughout the house, made sure all the doors were locked, and drove to Lee's Summit Medical Center to tend to Mom.

LESSON 7: Don't let denial fool you; be realistic with the situation.

It was a very quiet drive.

Fuck me. This is too much.

We arrived at the Lee's Summit Medical Center ER and found Mom unconscious, lying in an ER bed. The medical staff stabilized and sedated her to stop the seizures. When the doctor arrived, he asked all the basic questions, and I informed him of her situation (her complete you-aren't-gonna-believe-this situation). The doctor wanted to send her for a CT scan. Knowing she had just been in the sister hospital not more than three days prior, I informed him she just had a CT scan and told him it wasn't necessary.

Me: *"It's in her hospital records from Research just a few days ago."*
Doctor: *"It is protocol."*
Me: *"Fine, I would like a filet dinner please."*
Doctor: *"What do you mean?"*
Me: *"You are going to buy me a steak dinner because I am telling you, you will find nothing with a CT scan. She just had one within the last week. There is nothing wrong with her brain, this is something completely different."*

Yes, I did say that to him. For the last ten days, I had been in two different hospitals, meeting with different types of doctors, all to inform them about my Mom and what she was experiencing both emotionally and physically. Doesn't a sense of humor help in these situations? I was also ticked, yet again, that a physician wasn't listening to helpful, relevant information that I knew. Sure enough, the CT scan came back showing nothing.

Vindication! A small win.

Yet we still didn't know why this seizure occurred.

I did not get my steak dinner.

Unbeknownst to me, while I was checking Mom into the ER and filling out all the paperwork, Scott parked the car and made a phone call on my behalf. He reached out to our dear friend and college classmate, Steve, to give him a heads up on all the life events happening. Scott asked Steve to call me.

While waiting for the ER doctor to share the diagnosis, Steve called me. My face lit up when his cell phone number popped up, and I happily picked up the phone. His voice, his laughter, and his love for me were exactly what I needed at that moment. I am forever grateful for the distraction he gave me and the boost to my well-being with that one-single phone call. Friends, if you are reading this, and you know of someone who is having a life event, reach out to them, they need you. Be their distraction in a supportive loving way.

LESSON 8: Friends are important, and you still need to laugh.

For over a week, Mom was glacially slow to recover from this last seizure; it really whacked her out. When she did speak, it was sheer silliness that made no sense. She began talking about John, my dad, whom she divorced twenty-five years ago. After this seizure, she would not be the same. Honestly, she never truly regained her normal state of being. Her sharpness was gone. From her previous hospital stay five days before, they think (never confirmed) the seizures were a potential side effect of stopping one of her trigeminal neuralgia medications cold turkey, instead of weaning her off of it slowly. I later checked and found one of the side effects of stopping this medication—seizures. That night, Mom was admitted to Lee's Summit Medical Center.

Why didn't I ask more questions?
I can't take much more.

Let's hit the pause button and circle back to Walt at Research Medical Center, lying unconscious in an ICU bed on a ventilator.

His son Lynn was flying in from Salt Lake City to see him.

And now, I had a completely different mother to care for, lying in a bed at Lee's Summit Medical Center after a severe convulsive seizure.

LESSON 9: Just when you think you cannot take anymore, you find the strength to continue.

9

WHAT NOW? GET ORGANIZED
2012

Mercy, the last few days were a whirlwind of stress, dare I say, a tornado. It's time for me to take over and manage this new life situation we are all in. To this day, I can close my eyes and transcend back to Mom's hospital room on Mother's Day 2012, when Dr. Vincent shared the matter-of-fact diagnosis of dementia. I felt like I was floating above Mom's hospital bed, watching Dr. Vincent explain dementia to all of us. One of those surreal life moments.

I know it was Alzheimer's.

Sure, we had a dementia diagnosis, but what does it mean exactly? What do we do or not do? I wasn't prepared to ask questions; I had no clue what I should or shouldn't ask. I just accepted his words, with no questioning, which wasn't like me.

After Mom's recent seizure and realizing Walt would not recover, reality hit. I would be in charge. There was no discussion, it is just what happened. So, what to do? I found one of those black and white composition notebooks we all used in school. And I just started using it, writing in it, putting dates, and times and the many healthcare people that I spoke with in it. I kept records. I also used Google search to see what popped up related to dementia, Alzheimer's, and caregiving.

Naturally, I go to www.alz.org to devour all the information that I can get my hands on. Armed with my architectural background of problem-solving and project management skills, acquired over a thirty-year career, I knew I needed to educate myself. Knowledge is power, and I had so many questions. In architectural design school, professors taught us to think about several solutions before settling on the perfect one. We would stay up all hours of the night designing, pondering, and sketching until the perfect design solution made itself known. Now, I would apply the same problem-solving skills to Mom. I would read, talk to people, and Google the shit out of any scientific news article, blog, or whatever I could find to gain knowledge about the disease. I can deal with a situation once I gather all the knowledge to formulate a reasonable action plan.

LESSON 10: Find a notebook and use it.

- Create a question list for the next time you speak with the nurse or doctor.
- Glue or scotch tape the business cards you will collect in this new paper best friend.
- Write down the date, time, and person you spoke with, every time.
- Write down any knowledge or questions you share with the caregivers.
- Write down all the prescriptions your loved one is taking.
- Write down the pharmacy names and phone numbers.
- Write down the doctors' names and phone numbers.

- Write down all their friends and their phone numbers.
- Write down the names and phone numbers of their relatives.
- Write down the names and phone numbers of their clergy.
- Copies of driver's license.
- Copies of Social Security cards and numbers.
- Copies of insurance cards and phone numbers.
- Copies of Medicaid or Medicare cards.
- Get all the important items of your loved one's life.
- Add any pertinent milestone dates that could be of use.
- Gather any legal documents, if they have them: a durable power of attorney, last will, and loved one's wishes (these did not exist for me).

This notebook will become your beacon of sanity, accompanying you on your journey.

Just like American Express, don't leave home without it.

Below is a form letter I wrote and asked the nurses to keep in her chart. When Mom became anxious, they would hand her a copy of this letter in an attempt to remind her of what had happened.

Dear Mom -
Wednesday 9 May 2012 both of our worlds changed. Seeing you in the condition you were in at your house was shocking and scary at the same time.

I am very grateful Walt called when he did and shudder to think what would have happened to you if we did not take you to the emergency room when we did.

The next few days while in the hospital both of us witnessed you in various states of coherency. Both doctors agreed that your sodium level caused your confused mental state. Both doctors hoped when your sodium level came back within normal limits your solid mental state would return. What you are experiencing does not make you crazy. There is a chemical or neurological imbalance somewhere within your body and Dr Vincent needs to complete tests to determine the cause. Once the cause is determined, appropriate medicine can be prescribed to stabilize your condition. Again, you are not crazy, and I cannot imagine how strange all this must seem to you. I love you: know that. Walt loves you too!

Many of my friends my age has parents who are experiencing similar situations. Each mom or dad handles their condition differently, but what seems to be the hardest is when the parent thinks the child is being mean or doesn't love them. I need you to always remember I love you and want good things for you. I suggest you keep this letter handy as a reminder of my commitment to you.

I love you, Mom!
Sonya

10

WHICH HOSPITAL TO VISIT?
NOVEMBER 2012

Walt was at Research Medical Center on a ventilator. Mom was at Lee's Summit Medical Center in a comatose state, due to her most recent seizure. I was exhausted.

I can't make this up!

As anxious as I was for Lynn and his family to show up, it was somewhat of a relief for me. It gave me a respite from focusing on Walt and the ability to turn my full attention to Mom.

I empathized with Lynn's situation of receiving the dreaded phone call. As difficult as it was for me to make the call, it had to be even harder for him, knowing that when he arrived at the hospital, his father would not be conscious. He would not have the gift of saying a proper goodbye.

Those fourteen days became a rinse-and-repeat cycle full of anxiety, angst, and unknowns. My day consisted of waking up, getting dressed, touching base with work, driving to Research Medical Center, and checking in on Walt. Then I would drive to Lee's Summit Medical Center to be with Mom in hopes that today would be the day she would regain some form of consciousness. The most recent seizure truly kicked her butt.

Lynn stayed for one week and then returned home to Salt Lake City. Walt remained on the ventilator. Mom was released to the Pleasant Hill Rehabilitation Facility to regain her cognitive abilities from her last seizure. She was awake, she was somewhat mobile, and yet, not fully coherent.

During Lynn's time in Kansas City, he continued to ask questions about Mom and Walt to comprehend how this had happened without him knowing anything about it. The pleaser in me did my best to give comfort to Lynn during his time in Kansas City. He wanted to visit the farm and stay in Mom and Walt's farmhouse, frankly, because he didn't want to pay for a hotel. Because there had not been any financial planning, I needed to protect Mom and what was left of her future.

> *There is no way on earth I am letting you step foot inside that house. The only reason you want to see inside is to take anything valuable. No way.*

I did not want Lynn to have any access to the house. Sadly, I knew Walt had not long in this world. Mom would be all alone and whatever possessions in the house would be sold to pay for her long-term care. She needed the funds. I was not totally heartless. I knew enough from Mom as to which items had been in Walt's family. They would be returned to them in due time. I did not have the stamina to allow any of Walt's kids the ability to step foot in the farmhouse. Besides, there were so many spiders and dead mice in the basement. I used that little tidbit to my advantage. It was true.

Lynn: *"I spoke with Fred and learned dad sold one of his guns. Was money a problem?"*

Me: *"I have no idea. But I don't think so"*.
Lynn: *"Do you know if dad sold the family shotgun?"*
Me: *"I don't know."*
Lynn: *"Did dad sell his coin collection?"*
Me: *"I don't know."*

In crises, isn't it funny
what family members ask?

The fourteen days were up, and the day arrived when Walt's family had to make the decision. The hospital arranged a conference call, with a palliative care nurse joining us, to ask and answer questions. On the phone were Walt's son Lynn and Walt's brother Hal from Tucson. Scott and I were in attendance too. Mom was in Pleasant Hill Rehabilitation and was not on the phone due to her current mental state; her cognitive abilities had not returned.

LESSON 11: Have the discussion before you need to have the discussion.

This was a painful conference call. I felt helpless, sad, and defeated because I was being pushed into a corner without having the confidence to make the decision. None of us had had "the end-of-life talk" with a parent. I could hear the sadness in Lynn's voice. Walt's brother Hal wanted to ensure his brother was not in any pain.

Hal: *"What will happen to him once the tube is removed? Will he drown to death? Will he gasp for air? Will he be in pain? How do you know? This sounds so horrible."*

The palliative care nurse was empathetically wonderful. He reassured us that Walt was in no pain. He walked us through the scenarios, and based upon his knowledge and experience, what we could expect with each. During the conference call, I shared that I had finally found a DNR (do not resuscitate) that Walt and Mom had both signed a few years earlier through the VA. However, they never shared it with anyone but themselves, and they only gave each other the power to make life decisions!

LESSON 12: When you create a legally binding durable power of attorney document, ensure you also grant power to someone other than your significant other and give them copies.

The collective decision was made to remove the ventilator and place Walt in palliative care within the hospital. At this point in healthcare, hospice had leaped mainstream, and Research Medical Center had partnered with VITAS Healthcare to create a hospice unit on the sixth floor. It was still a hospital wing, but the interior designer created a calming presence within this unit by using soft lighting with a soothing color scheme. It was a quiet place for reflection for those visiting their loved ones. The palliative care nurse assured us he would be watched closely, with pain management first and foremost. He would be made comfortable.

Lynn: *"How long will this take?"*

Over the next few days, my focus returned to work as there was nothing more I could do for Walt or Mom. Time was in control. As difficult as it was, we all would wait.

Thursday morning I was at work, walking through a tenant space, and discussing spatial designs with my boss. My cell phone buzzed, and I saw the hospital number. With a bit of gloom, I answered the call. It was the hospice nurse informing me that Walt had passed away. Walt's mother was by his side that morning. Thank goodness someone was with him.

I asked the hospice nurse to call John Dickey, with Stanley-Dickey Funeral Home, to collect Walt. The previous weekend, Scott and I had met with John to pick out Walt's casket and make a few of the arrangements. Mom was still in a noncoherent state, and I knew we needed to postpone Walt's funeral until Mom recovered. You see, decades ago, Mom's sister Georgia had been in a horrific car accident, which killed her husband. Even as a little kid, I remembered Mom flying to California to attend the funeral. Because of the accident, Georgia was in the hospital and could not attend her own husband's funeral. When she woke up and recovered, it was horrible for her. That scenario remained with me all these years, and I didn't want Mom to experience what Aunt Georgia had. I knew Mom needed to say her goodbyes to Walter.

We had not settled on any of the dates, and due to Mom's current state of being, I was not in any hurry to bury Walt. I had asked for the funeral home to put Walt in storage. Selfishly, I needed a break.

11

FAMILY DYNAMICS

Everyone has a family. I would like to introduce you to mine. Both of my parents grew up poor in rural Kentucky. Behavioralists say our learned behavior comes from our parents. Well, Mom and dad learned from their parents both good and bad. Both of their parents had a tough life, a hard time putting food on the table and raising kids. Farming and gardening were a necessity for both families to ensure there was food, not necessarily plenty, but food.

Dad's parents, Harris and Lillian Likins, were dairy farmers living in tiny Caneyville, Kentucky, population 500. They raised four kids: Betty, Patsy, my dad, and Joe Mike. Grandma and Grandpa Likins were prime examples of unhappy behavior. Grandpa Harris was a mean person, and yours truly was frightened of this man! I wanted nothing to do with him. Grandma Lillian dutifully took care of Harris. She was a soft-spoken woman and did her best to bring light-heartedness into the family. Yet the burden of living with an unhappy man showed itself on her face. When Bob and I were around, she worked to shield us from Grandpa Harris. When our family visited them on the Caneyville farm, I witnessed my parents walking on eggshells, trying to not piss off Harris. It was such strange behavior to watch grown adults act like me who was a child. Not much love was being spread around the Likins family.

Dad learned hardship with no love. So sad.

Dad's childhood was one of long, hard days of farm work, then he'd get up and do it all over again.

Mom and dad met at Caneyville High School. I want to believe the beginning of their relationship was filled with love and optimism, two young adults wanting more than their parents had. They both wanted to leave Grayson County, Kentucky, and explore. They wanted more. Dad enlisted in the Army, and off he went to Germany to serve his country. At the time, the GI bill provided hope to many young women and men. If they served their country, their country would pay them back to attend college. After the Army, he used the GI bill to pay for his college education at Western Kentucky. I believe it is still the best government program created.

While cleaning out Mom and Walt's house, I discovered a box filled with dad's report cards from college. College was not easy for dad; he struggled to achieve passing grades, but graduate he did. Mom and dad eloped to Robertson County, Tennessee one weekend in March 1957. Their first child, my brother Bob, arrived within a year. It was a struggle for all of them. Both Mom and dad worked odd jobs to support the family, with the emphasis on dad gaining an education to elevate themselves out of the lower class. Mom and dad knew they wanted a different life, not only for themselves but for their children. For the most part, they did a good job ensuring both Bob and I had a college education to gain better jobs than they had.

Growing up, how do you tell someone that you were frightened of your own father? I never knew which dad would be around. Was it Social John? Or would it be Mean

John? Knowing if I did the right kid things, such as keeping a clean room, doing homework, getting straight A's, just laying low, and being a good kid, I would not feel the physical or emotional wrath of John. Unfortunately, my brother felt the sometimes physical wrath of our dad a little too much. I just couldn't understand why dad was always so angry and unhappy. He learned from his parents.

Mom was born in Shrewsbury, Kentucky, to Pete and Bessie Davis. Grandpa Pete was a carpenter and over the years helped build many homes and buildings, while Grandma Bess tended to the house, garden, and family. Grandma and Grandpa Davis were prime examples of loving, happy behavior. They were just adorable together—he in his blue jean overalls, faded and worn from work, and her in her housecoat and slippers she wore every day. Mom was the fifth child of what would eventually be twelve children altogether—nine girls and three boys. Mom would tell me the family was dirt poor growing up, but there was always laughter, hugs, stories, and some food. All the kids participated in working around the tiny house and country farm to ensure chores were done. From a very young age, Pete and Bessie instilled a work ethic for all their children. Mom knew hard work, and it didn't bother her; she thrived working. Growing up in the country was tough for all the kids. They all shared in the chores: tending to the garden, feeding the animals, preparing meals, washing clothes, and taking turns at the outhouse. Five kids under one roof, sharing beds, and living life.

As a kid, I loved visiting Grandma and Grandpa Davis in their tiny brick suburban home in Louisville. They would greet our family with love, hugs, and desserts! Sure, my aunts and uncles squabbled, yet it was always in loving, good fun. Grandma loved the garden and their carport, which the family used as a covered patio, surrounded by elephant ear plants. As a five-year-old running around the back yard, those large green leaves were fascinating to me. So much love existed within the Davis family.

Mom learned to laugh and love. So grateful.

After graduation, dad landed a job with International Harvester. After my birth in Lexington, the family moved to Louisville briefly and then to Bucyrus, Ohio. Moving would be repeated over and over. His job provided a solid income for us as a family and gave my parents the catapult from rural poverty life to lower-middle-class America. Every two years we moved around Ohio; Bucyrus, Columbus; Wilmington; and finally Marysville.

From 1976 to 1978, I went from a teenager to a young adult. I watched my parents' marriage deteriorate, and my dad devolved into his father Harris. I would love to paint a rosy picture of a happy marriage, but I cannot. Brother Bob was enrolled at Ohio State University, studying mechanical engineering. Dad worked for International Harvester, Mom worked for Deluxe checks, and I was a dorky kid in fifth grade. Bob would visit us on the weekends, and it was the highlight of my week. We were seven years apart, and I worshipped my big brother. In my eyes, he could do no wrong. For our parents, well, our dad, it was a different story.

Bob gave me my first bicycle—a pink bike with a matching pink banana seat. He taught me how to ride a bike, not dad. When we lived in Columbus, that first bike ride at the age of six, without training wheels, was led by my brother. I followed behind him riding through the subdivision. I remember my focus on balance, looking ahead, concentrating on him and the moves he made. That was until I turned my head to look at the new houses under construction. Within seconds, the bike veered toward the concrete curb. There was nothing I could do but accept my fate in a crash. Front tire, meet curb. I flew off the bike and landed with a thud. My lip hit the pavement and immediately started bleeding, and I started to cry. It wasn't so much that it hurt, I was just shocked. Bob scooped me up and ran me back to the house, which was just a block away. My lip swelled, and not in a good Botox way, but a puffy scab way. A few days later, I started kindergarten. Maybe that experience of starting kindergarten with a fat, puffy, scabby lip helped me build character!

I would like to think that.

When dad received another job opportunity to leave Ohio and move to Kansas City in 1978, my parents said yes. It was an opportunity dad had to take. Even if it meant leaving Bob in Ohio. He and Faith, his high school sweetheart, were definitely an item. It was a forgone conclusion they would wed. Bob was attending college, and his many friends were there too. His life was in Ohio, not Kansas.

Bob helped us move to Kansas and settle in. I have fond memories of driving Interstate 70 from Ohio to Kansas and playing alphabet bingo. (At least, that's what we called it.) Who knew that Missouri had a Z highway? I won that game!

Bob's visits to Kansas were over the usual holidays. On occasion, we would drive back to Ohio to visit as well. When we moved to Kansas, I was in eighth grade and a total nerd. Starting a new school at that age builds character. It also introduced me to my oldest friend David Allen.

As Bob's baby sister, I was sad, heartbroken, and lost without my brother. He was always there for me, and I knew I could count on him. Sure, we talked on the phone, yet it wasn't the same. He had always watched over me.

As time passed with Bob in Ohio, and the three of us in Kansas, it was only natural we would grow distant. Mom was very grateful that Al and Eleanor Baxter, Faith's parents, completely welcomed Bob into their family. Eventually, Bob and Faith wed and are currently living happily ever after in Ohio, close to their two daughters Katie and Maggie, and their families. Mom was so proud of Bob and Faith, and, oh, those granddaughters were her pride and joy. She loved each of them dearly and welcomed all forms of engagement sent her way.

Throughout Mom's dementia journey, Bob and I would text, email, and chat on occasion. From my side, it was just the right amount of touch points to keep him in the loop on Mom's health. When Mom would have her bout of OCD phone calls, Bob would call to share the conversation, or rather the panic in Mom's voice. I am grateful we were both aligned on the quality of life we wanted for our mother. We both knew what she wanted and didn't.

Bob had experienced his in-laws, Al and Eleanor Baxter, with their age-related illnesses. When both were experiencing their respective issues, Bob and I would have amazing vulnerable conversations about end-of-life care and what we would want. We both agreed how painfully helpless you feel watching your loved one struggle when you know they will not get better. We would talk about what quality of life meant to each of us and at what point would we say, "Enough." When we might say, "I am ready to let go and elevate to another dimension." (Side note, read Stephen King's *Elevation*. Excellent read.)

We might go about it by asking ourselves:

- What do we want?
- What don't we want?
- When is enough, enough? What are the parameters?
- Would we relocate to another state where assisted suicide is legal?

- Would we sit outside in the cold of winter and freeze to death?
- Where would we want to experience our last breath? In a hospital? On a beach? In the mountains?

I am a firm believer that God gave us free will. It is our life; we make our choices. We get to choose what is right for us. Unselfish love is supporting one another in those choices and fulfilling those wishes.

LESSON 13: Speak to your family, your entire family, about your wishes. Don't be shy. Let them know exactly what you do and don't want. Let them know your definition of quality of life.

Mom had experienced the pain of watching her father struggle with strokes and hospitalization. Her own aging mother Bessie went through not talking, not eating, not walking, and being confined to a bed. It broke Mom's heart. She did not want the same path for herself. Her quality of life was everything.

At a recent wedding reception, the father of the bride gave a glorious, loving, sincere toast to his daughter and son-in-law. It was filled with love, and he had put work into creating the perfect toast. As I sat there and listened to his words, I began to cry, not only for the love this father publicly exhibited towards his daughter but because I didn't have this experience myself.

While writing this book, our dad became ill, moved into a nursing home, and passed away in May 2022. Bob took care of dad who was living back in Caneyville. Just like Mom and

Walt, Bob had his own share of issues to deal with, such as no will, no power of attorney, and limited funds. Folks, if you don't know anything about probate, it is no fun dealing with it.

One of the many reasons I cried during the father of the bride's toast, my father never would have taken the time to write a toast or tell me that he loved me. He had become an angry selfish man, just like his father. So, when Mom told me that night, so many years ago, she started the divorce process, I was so happy for both of us. Thank you, Mom.

12

HOW TO TELL MOM?
NOVEMBER 2012

While Walt's family had decided to take him off the ventilator, Mom was in Lee's Summit Medical Center recovering from her most recent seizure. She stayed at Lee's Summit for five days, then was released to the Pleasant Hill Health and Rehabilitation Center where she would spend the rest of the year recovering. That name always made me chuckle as it imposed an idyllic way of life. It wasn't the prettiest of places, but the staff was good. Or so I thought.

Mom was a challenge for everyone. She was strong, stubborn, and mobile. Because of her recent seizures, the healthcare industry considered her a "fall risk." She was not. As a matter of facility protocol, they placed her in a wheelchair with an alarm. When she stood up, the alarm went off. Did I mention Mom never wanted to be a burden to anyone? Because of the alarm on the wheelchair, she quickly learned not to stand up, even if she needed to go to the bathroom!

Which means she held her urine.

One evening, I received a call from the rehabilitation facility explaining that Mom was having a tantrum in the middle of the hallway. She was screaming, yelling, ripping her clothes off, and not allowing anyone near her. They called an ambulance to escort Mom back to the Lee's Summit Medical Center ER. We were familiar with this ER because we had been there only a few days before. Scott and I hopped into our car and drove toward the ER.

Weren't we just there?

By now, I know the drill. She is checked in, doctors and nurses go through their normal routines, and we are called in for the diagnosis. She has a UTI (urinary tract infection). I will soon learn that UTIs create havoc in people! Remember I shared with you the alarm on Mom's wheelchair to discourage her from standing up? Remember how I shared Mom didn't want to be a burden? Add those two together, and she just sat in the wheelchair holding her urine. When she felt the urge to urinate, Mom would stand up. By standing up, the alarm on her wheelchair would sound. She didn't like the sound and realized if she sat down, no more sound. She didn't want to be a burden, so she promptly sat down. By holding her urine for a long time, she contracted a UTI. When the nurse finally drained her bladder, there was more than one liter of fluid!

At this point, I was learning to ask all sorts of questions. There were always different points of view, and I did my best to gather information. The following day, I had a phone call with the urologist, and it wasn't the best.

The urologist shared that, in his experience, a person with a bladder distension of that magnitude would have a permanent problem and the solution is to install a suprapubic catheter.

A what?

A suprapubic catheter is a hollow, flexible tube that is used to drain urine from the bladder. It is inserted into the bladder through a cut in the abdomen, a few inches below the navel. The catheter connects to a collection bag, which becomes an added appendage to the patient. I couldn't imagine Mom living with one of these for the rest of her life. She would pick at it and play with it. It would bother anyone.

I had conducted a bit of due diligence before the urology call, as I knew the catheter was an option. I learned someone could recover from infrequent UTIs. My due diligence included calling my niece, Dr. Maggie, and asking about all the possibilities to remedy Mom's bladder. I shared with the urologist the recent life events that had led Mom to this point. I shared Walt's death, her not wanting to be a burden, the alarm on the wheelchair, and her recent seizures. I did all I could to convey to the urologist her extraordinary life conditions. This was a woman who would bounce back; I needed the urologist to understand that.

> **Dr. Moosehead:** *"In my thirty-six years as a urologist, I have never seen anyone recover from this much bladder distension. Her bladder will not recover, and we need to install the permanent catheter."*
> **Me:** *"You haven't met my mother."*

LESSON 14: Be the advocate! Trust buy verify!

The doctor left her urinary catheter in, along with the urine bag strapped to her leg. The intent was to give Mom time to heal and take a wait-and-see approach to her bladder issue. Mom returned to Pleasant Hill Health and Rehabilitation Facility for another week to recover from the UTI. During this time, her cognitive abilities slowly came back. I don't know how to say it, but she was whacked out from the UTI, and to witness a loved one in that state of mind is so very hard. One memory I have, she was in a wheelchair at the lunch table eating a roll like a squirrel. She had a faraway look in her eye and her only focus was to hold the roll and take little bites while extremely focused on chewing. This was happening at the same time I needed to tell her about Walt's death. That was another hard conversation to have.

How do I tell Mom that Walt has died?

Mom had been in and out of the hospital for over two weeks since Walt was placed on a ventilator. She had been unconscious when Walt died. Her last memory, if she had one, was of Walt lying in an ICU bed with the tube down his throat. She was now staying in another strange place, where she knew no one, and her daughter was the one telling her that her Walter had passed away.

LESSON 15: One doesn't know where strength or sheer willpower comes from. Somehow, we find it.

Ironically, of all my memories of her dementia journey, this one, telling my Mom about Walt's passing, I have no recollection. I know Scott and I were together in the common area of her current facility, telling her the news. I truly do not know if she understood me, yet I know she had some conscious understanding even while recovering from her UTI.

Mom recovered fully from her UTI, and all catheters were removed.

The funeral home put Walt in cold storage for a week. I decided to wait for Mom to recover and say her goodbyes, then we would have a funeral for Walt. Thankfully, Mom and Walt had made a few burial arrangements. They had picked out their burial plot in the local Pleasant Hill Cemetery and were to be laid to rest alongside Walt's family: mother, father, siblings, and cousins. The gravestone was installed, awaiting Mom and Walt's final engraved dates.

Looking back, Mom endured the Sunday four-hour visitation, greeting, and hugging everyone with her bladder bag strapped to her leg, hidden underneath her pants. She was Social Mom with smiles, love, and laughter. She sat in a chair next to Walt's open casket, fondly looking at him, kissing him, and touching his hands. Oh, she missed him. Considering everything she had been through, she rallied. Walt would have been humbled by the show of support and love for him, but more importantly, for his Deanie. The local Shriners performed a service ritual after the visitation was over to pay their respects to Walter and his years of service to both the country and the Shriners.

I am very grateful for my Aunt Susan and Uncle Steve who made the journey from Louisville, Kentucky, to be with Mom for Walt's funeral. It was wonderful to have a bit of respite with my family present. I needed to laugh. And Mom loved the attention too!

Walt's funeral service was held at their tiny church—Big Creek Baptist Church. Pastor Todd MacLean performed the simple, heartfelt service as he knew both Mom and Walt well. We sang a few hymns, and I delivered Walt's eulogy on Mom's behalf.

Walt's Eulogy:

"How do we measure a life? Some say it's by the size of one's bank account. Others believe it's how they live their life. Still others believe it is the number of friends and family surrounding them during a challenging life experience, whether it's a birth of twins, an illness, or death.

I think each of us can say, and believe, Walt Mitchell lived a full life.

We ask you to not mourn the loss but to remember and celebrate his life. Remember the things that mattered most to Walt: family, church, service to country, friends, birds, and gardening, a good hug, and the telling of a good story. We are all blessed and richer for having Walt in our lives.

Walt loved Dean. As the story goes, they are Lucky Ducks to have found each other and shared twenty wonderful years. It has been an amazing experience to watch them, giddy with new love. They loved each other's company and had the ability to sit and talk for hours. Still not sure how that is possible, but they did it.

Thank you, everyone, for your love, support, and prayers during the last four weeks. Both Walt and Dean needed you, and you were there for them: the children, grandchildren, and great-grandchildren. Thank you very much.

After the church service, the casket was loaded into the back of the hearse, and we drove to the cemetery located a few blocks away. Pastor Todd MacLean said a few graveside words. The local VFW sent soldiers to present Mom with a folded American flag and Walt with a patriotic five-gun salute. A humbling moment for all those in attendance. The casket was lowered, and we all said our goodbyes. Everyone left the cemetery and went in separate directions.

Funeral complete: check.
Walt buried: check.
Mom back to Pleasant Hill Rehabilitation Facility: check.
We go home: check.

13

DEAN, DEAN THE BUTTERBEAN

We all say and believe our parents are the best. Yes, my Mom was the best. She had the biggest heart and loved other people. She would do anything for anyone. She loved pleasing others and seeing people happy. She saw the goodness in everyone.

She grew up in a large family, and they didn't have much. Her parents, Bess and Pete Davis, obviously loved each other; they had twelve kids under one roof. Mom and her sisters were relegated to cooking, cleaning, and helping on the family farm by gardening or tending to farm animals. Mom shared her reasons for not liking dogs. When feeding the hunting dogs on the farm, they would jump on her, and that was not right in her estimation.

Mom never learned to swim, yet she wanted to make sure Bob and I knew how to swim. In the summer months growing up, she would take us to early morning swim lessons at the neighborhood public pool. Ironically, I learned to dog paddle and float, but I never mastered the breaststroke until I signed up for adult swim lessons this last year.

Living in rural western Kentucky, she and her siblings attended a one-room schoolhouse. As the county's population grew, a high school was ultimately built, and she and her classmates would graduate from Caneyville High School, class of 1956. She and her best friend Verna Jean moved to Louisville and lived in a shared apartment. They were both telephone switchboard operators. I have a black and white photo image of Mom wearing headphones with wires connected to the switchboard. She's neatly dressed in a skirt, sweater, black kitten-heeled pumps, pearls, and her hair just so, and it makes me smile. She worked hard and saved every penny to buy the things her parents could not afford.

Back in the day, purchasing items on layaway was the method to accumulate household items. As I cleaned out the farmhouse, I would discover the many treasures she had purchased during those years living with Verna Jean; she just couldn't part with them. These porcelain figurine items had been in our house for as long as I could remember. There was the trio of cows, a momma cat, and her two kittens, and two Asian boy and girl figurines—for which Mom would proudly remind me of the "Made in Japan" stamp on the bottom.

When she baked homemade pies, she took the extra pie crust and rolled it out. She would cut the pie crusts into strips, sprinkle them with sugar and cinnamon, then bake them. So yummy!

Mom always worked. During my early grade school years, she worked part-time to ensure she was home when the school bus dropped me off. As I grew up, she took on a full-time job, which coincided with Bob attending university. I know my parents struggled with money, and I am confident Mom worked to pay for Bob's college and to give us the extras in life—dinners out, new clothes, or household upgrades. She instilled in my brother and me a driven work ethic. A little hard work never hurt anyone.

Her large family, the Davis family, had epic family reunions. All the women would cook, and the amount of food at these reunions was insane. There were all sorts of casseroles, Jell-O salads, potato salads, coleslaw, hot dogs, burgers, cakes, pies, cookies, sweet tea, and sodas. The girls would share the latest National Enquirer gossip, and the room was filled with laughter. When the topic would bleed over to Dolly Parton and Porter Wagner, watch out, these ladies were serious about those entertainers. The Johnny Cash and June Carter Cash tumultuous relationship would cause a ruckus with them. Oh, and then there was Elvis and his eating habits, drug habits, and his relationship with Priscilla. I would sit on the stool in the corner and listen with delight. I couldn't get enough.

Mom and dad married at a very early age, and Bob was born shortly after. I know the early years of their marriage were difficult and they were poor. Dad attended Western Kentucky University, and Mom worked full-time as a telephone operator to make ends meet. Dad had a part-time job while attending college. I came along seven years after my brother.

Neither of them talked about the early years much.

As a child, I never wanted for anything. Mom made sure Bob and I had what we needed. Mom knew education was key, and she was darn sure the both of us would have a college degree. During my last year in college, Mom worked three jobs to provide for the two of us. After she divorced dad, dad would not pay anymore. She was determined to keep the house and pay for my last year of college. I am so very grateful.

Mom's given name was Willa Dean Davis. She always went by Dean, even as a kid. It was during her school years in the Caneyville school system that she acquired the nickname of Dean, Dean the Butterbean. It fit her.

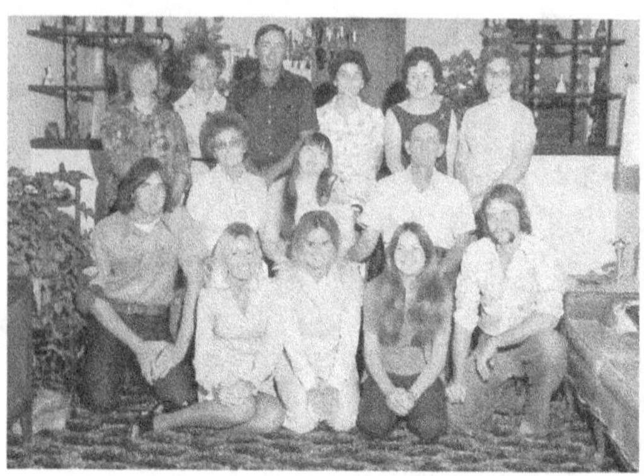

Back row, left to right: Sherry, Mom, Charles, Urma,
Georgia, Verde. Middle row, left to right: David,
Grandma Davis, Diane, Grandpa Davis. Front row, left
to right: Barbara, June Dale, Susan, Eddie

14

MOM'S NEW HOME
JANUARY 2013

After Walt's funeral, Mom stayed at Pleasant Hill Health and Rehabilitation through December 2012 under the coverage of skilled nursing care. She had daily PT/OT sessions and wandered the halls as much as the staff would allow. Each day she healed toward her Normal Mom self. She continued to wear the bladder bag, and thankfully, her bladder quickly returned to normal. Within a few weeks, the appendage came off and she was free and clear with no catheter! I was very clear, no more alarms; let her walk and be mobile. I don't think they liked that. Scott and I visited her every weekend to take her out and about for a cheeseburger. Fortunately, Pleasant Hill had a McDonald's.

While Mom was recovering, I had been researching living facilities for her while dealing with all the financial and insurance challenges that were coming into play from Walt's passing and their farm. Bob, Scott, and I decided to keep Mom close to her home area of Pleasant Hill in hopes that the friends she and Walt had made would visit her. This decision left us with one option: Foxwood Springs in Raymore, Missouri. Foxwood Springs was a leisurely twenty-minute car ride, through the countryside, from their tiny town of Pleasant Hill, Missouri. Over the years, Foxwood Springs has grown into a nice retirement compound. They have single-family homes, a rehabilitation unit, a two-story apartment complex, an assisted living wing, and a memory care wing. The trend in senior living is one-stop shopping (age-in-place, or as I call it, Hotel California. As the Eagles song goes, "You can check out anytime you like, but you can never leave."

In January 2013, we moved Mom into a studio located directly adjacent to the nurses' station, and that opened onto the shared living/dining area. I felt it was ideal for Mom, the social butterfly. I quickly learned it was too noisy for her.

She hated living at Foxwood for the first month. Hated it. Slowly, she made friends and adapted to her new environment. Like a light switch that flipped on, all the drama calmed down for a bit, and each of us began adapting to our new normal.

I did my best to call her every couple of days to check-in. Every weekend, I made the sixty-minute round-trip drive to see her. The visit typically included lunch out and a trip through Walmart to pick up anything she thought she needed.

Growing up, it was not uncommon for me to return home from school and find new clothes lying on my bed. When Mom shopped for either of us, it was a complete ensemble of a shirt and pants that blended perfectly together. Mom had style, and she ensured her kids looked good. Our beds would be made, and she would arrange our new clothes on the bed, just so. Typically, placed at an angle on the bed, with the sleeve of the shirt folded to look like the shirt's hand was on the hip of the pants. For me, I would get appropriate jewelry to complete my ensemble. That surprising thrill of walking into my bedroom and seeing new clothes on my bed still brings a smile to my face. For Mom's new place at Foxwood, I wanted her to experience that same thrill.

When Scott and I moved Mom into Foxwood, her room was all laid out and waiting for her:

- Full size bed with a new bedspread, sheets, and pillows
- Family photos on the wall, specifically of Walt
- Art on the wall
- A telephone with a large font printed telephone list of key friends and family phone numbers
- A new TV with remote control and large font printed instructions
- Her favorite orange recliner, side table, and reading lamp
- New window treatments over the bay window
- New bath towels
- New toothbrush and toothpaste
- New makeup
- Hand lotion
- A digital clock
- Her comb and hairbrush
- A small, magnified makeup mirror
- Clothes and shoes in the closet
- Socks and underwear folded and placed in the chest of drawers
- All clothing with name labels ironed into them
- Werther's candy, her favorite

Everything I had read online about dementia informed me to keep her room minimal; clutter was a bad thing. It looked sparse, but I knew it was the best for her. My normal was not her normal.

With lots of trepidation, Scott and I escorted Mom to Foxwood and walked her to her new room. It had been a bit shy of forty-five days since her world was turned upside down with Walt's illness, death, and funeral, her seizures, and

UTI. This would be her new home. The friendly staff greeted us and welcomed Mom with such excitement and care. It was so sweet to watch them interact with her. She beamed with excitement seeing all her things again. The nostalgic familiarity was overwhelming for her. For me, it brought relief and peace.

After all the antics over the last two months, I left Foxwood that day with a huge weight off my shoulders. Mom was settled in a safe place surrounded by people who would care for and grow to love her. I knew that, yet I was emotionally filled with guilt. There's a guilt about leaving a parent behind in a strange place. Logic told me it was the right thing to do, but my heart ached that I just couldn't be her daily full-time caregiver.

She will be okay.
Oh, the guilt.

15

ROAD TRIP WITH MOM

2013

By now, you are probably at the point in this read, where you are shaking your head and thinking I am looney. Or shame on me for not having more patience with Mom. Well, you are right.

The story I'm about to share paints me in a not-so-great light.

Maggie and Tim's wedding was planned for Saturday, February 2, 2013, in Deer Creek State Park, an hour southwest of Columbus, Ohio. Even with whatever dementia fog Mom was living in, she knew the wedding was happening and wondered how she was going to get there! *"Sonya, when is the wedding and how will we get there?"* Just like a five-year-old asking, "Why," this was her mantra.

As Mom had settled into her new home at Foxwood Springs, the telephone became her lifeline, no matter what time of day.

Maggie was the youngest of her two granddaughters. The oldest was Katie, who had married Arnold a few years before. Mom loved her only grandchildren and would do anything to be a part of their lives. Every year, Mom would find each of them their porcelain birthday girl figurine with the number representing that year's age and send it to them. Goofy as it was, there was so much love that went into finding those birthday figurines and sending them to her granddaughters. Mom would never say it, but living so far away from them was hard for her; she would have loved being part of their lives a bit more.

A week before the nuptials, yours truly had undergone a partial hysterectomy to resolve health issues. I was tired, sore, and couldn't lift anything. Which left the burden falling on Scott for our upcoming travel adventure. I was still healing, and Mom did not know about my surgery.

I didn't need to burden her
with my issues. Did I?

Thursday night in Kansas City, we drove to pick her up and have her spend the night with us. We thought it would make it easier for the next day of air travel. That night, we had a simple home-cooked meal so we could all go to bed early. Tomorrow was a big day of travel!

For many reasons, Scott and I did not have children, and I watched with wonder at the parents of challenging kids. How do they do it? I felt like a parent that entire trip. I was watching Mom's every move, making sure she picked up her feet, watching her fixation on shiny objects (small children and shiny signs in the airport), and ultimately, not bumping into anyone or falling. As we walked through Midway International Airport, she wasn't doing the best job of picking up her feet. She was shuffling a bit too much, and I worried about her balance.

Scott: *"Pick up your feet, Deanie!"*

She immediately started marching and raising her feet. Clunk, clunk, clunk—like a horse. Internally, I was sadly laughing. I guess the new K-Swiss shoes did not agree with her after all.

The other challenge with Mom was her fixation with young children. She had no fear of walking up to a small child and touching them, without any permission from a parent. I am grateful for the parents who understood. Of course, she would not harm any child, but did the parent know that?

Me: *"Mom, how about a McDonald's cheeseburger for lunch?"*
Mom: *"That sounds perfect!"*

One McDonald's cheeseburger (with ketchup only), fries, and a small Coke coming up. Mom did not need to be fed; she was capable. She would take the cheeseburger and remove all the extra bun/breading around the edges before eating it.

Mmmm...I do that too.

Small win—a McDonald's meal.

At this point in the day, I was tired after answering the same questions repeatedly, being on point to ensure her safety, and healing from my surgery. I am so very grateful for Scott's patience.

Me: *"Scott, I need a bit of reprieve. Are you okay with me walking around a bit before we board the plane to Columbus?"*
Scott: *"Sure."*

I just needed fifteen minutes of quiet time; no questions, no worries. Selfishly, I needed my time.

One more task before boarding, though: *"Mom, let's go to the bathroom."*

Off we go to the bathroom marching with clunking feet. March, clunk, march, clunk.

Fortunately, the flight from Chicago to Columbus was simple. At this point, she took direction well. She still had not fully recovered from her seizure a few months before and she was sad. She missed her Walt. Our conversation on the plane was meant to be entertaining for her. We talked about Bob, the granddaughters, Walt, and all the good times they had together. We did our best to remind her of all the good she had experienced. Essentially, we had the same conversations three or four times during the flight. If anyone is a fan of *50 First Dates*, rest assured the "Ten Second Tom" character was alive and well living within my Mom.

After landing, we clunked to the bathroom, baggage claim, and rental car counter. Loaded up, we headed to Deer Creek State Park for the weekend wedding festivities.

> **Mom:** *"Where are we? Where are we going? How much longer? Are we there yet? Why are we here? Who will we see? Will we see Bob?"* 1, 2, 3, 4, 5, 6, 7, 8, 9, 10...*"Where are we?"*

This was her world, and we were living in it. After a seventy-minute drive that felt like four hours, we arrived at our destination—Deer Creek State Park. A sense of relief washed over all of us.

Bob greeted us, and it was awesome for her. Selfishly, me too. My brother is a good soul and, as the first born, holds a special place in Mom's heart. She lit up seeing his face. Instantly, it warmed my heart and made the challenges of the day melt away. Selfishly, I was glad others were around to assist in entertaining Mom. I needed this after being on point since Walt's hospitalization last October, a mere four months ago.

We asked for adjoining rooms to keep a safe eye on Mom.

With her help, we unpacked her tiny green suitcase, hung up her clothes, and placed her toiletries in the bathroom—laid out on a towel—just the way she liked it. Through trial and error, and as Mom changed, we found it best to lay her toiletries out on a towel for her to see them easily. This way she would not need to dig through a drawer. Essentially, if she could find her toothbrush, toothpaste, and comb, it would be easier for her to remember to use them.

In another life, Mom would have had her entire makeup collection with her. Now, she needed only a few hygiene necessities: a comb, toothbrush, toothpaste, lipstick, deodorant, and face moisturizer. She didn't ask for anything more.

After a brief nap for all of us, we dressed to head to a private dining room at the lodge for the rehearsal dinner. I would be lying if I said my anxiety level was low; it was high because I didn't know which Mom would show up. Luckily, we all got to see Social Mom. She had a great evening chatting with the granddaughters, Maggie and Katie, as well as Bob, and his wife Faith, and all the Baxter family (Faith's family). Mom laughed and joked and reminisced about many events, some she remembered and some she did not. But you would never know it; she had developed the skill of smiling, agreeing, and being cagey. I don't mean cagey as in true manipulative deception, but rather, cagey as in saying yes and nodding just enough so you wouldn't challenge her or ask, *"Do you really remember that?"*

The rehearsal dinner was a nice evening of laughter and fun for all. We all went to bed early that night because the next day was the wedding of Maggie and Tim.

The big day was here, and it was going to be a fun day for all parties. Mom woke up early and, bless her heart, she quietly got dressed and waited for us to wake up and take her to breakfast. I texted Bob to ask if he would take Mom to breakfast and we would join them in a bit. Mom was thrilled to spend time with her son!

Scott and I headed to the breakfast room to meet them. As we sat down, my brother's glance met mine. His eyes said it all, "Where is the Mom I know?" We sat at the table and talked. Reminiscing of all things silly, previous weddings, current job updates, current events, and the wedding of the day. It was early in the morning and Mom was engaged. After breakfast, we walked around a bit, assisted Maggie and Katie with decorating for the wedding and enjoying each other's company.

As we left breakfast, I noticed an older guy checking into the lodge. It was my dad John. I didn't know Maggie had invited him to the wedding. This wasn't my wedding, it was theirs.

Really? Why?

It's not so much about me, truly; I couldn't care less. It was about Mom and her mental stability. Their marriage was not a happy one, and I did not want the sight of him to upset her. Yes, I was being overprotective.

Time got away from me that morning, and we had to rush back to our rooms to change clothes for the wedding ceremony. We got Mom dressed, me dressed, and we rushed back upstairs to the mezzanine just in time to be seated before the wedding started. Tim and Maggie said their "I do's" and twenty-minutes later were pronounced husband and wife. The wedding was simple and sweet, perfect for them. During the wedding, I glanced over at Mom, seated in her best jacket, blouse, and dress pants,

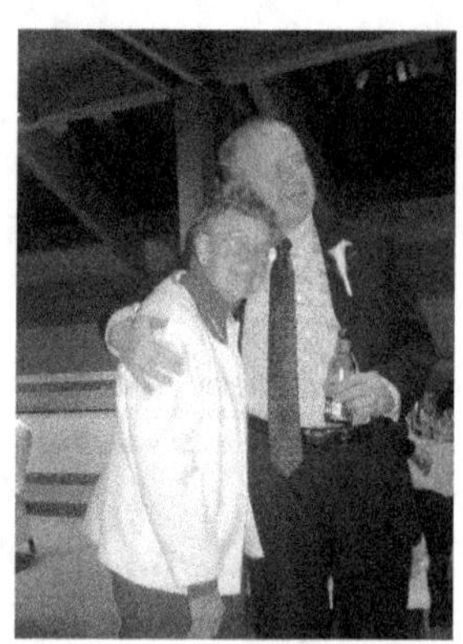

Mom and brother Bob

complete with a necklace and matching earrings, and with her Mom hair just so. Her eyes were glued on the happy couple; she was beaming. That moment, that smile, was all the love one can imagine projecting from one human to another; the love in her eyes for them made the trip.

LESSON 16: Cherish the little things in life and be present.

The reception began immediately after the ceremony. The guests shifted to their tables, and the DJ cranked up the tunes. Let the party begin!

Mom enjoyed sitting at the table and soaking it all in. She would lean over and ask me, *"Who is that person?"* All of Faith's family made it a point to speak with her and engage with her. Mom met everyone with a smile and polite conversation. I am sure she remembered most, yet I will never know for sure. Frankly, it doesn't matter. She was happy. Mom did catch a glimpse of her ex-husband in the crowd. She asked, *"Why is he here? Who invited him? Why would anyone invite him?"* Scott and I quickly went into redirection mode with her. This is a skill we had begun to master. Scott was much better at it than I was; I had too much emotional baggage hanging over my head to think clearly at times when it came to Mom.

As the reception started to wind down, I was exhausted and ready for bed. Mom was too. We walked back to our adjoining rooms. I helped Mom get ready for bed.

Me: *"Mom, time to get into our jammies. Mom, have you brushed your teeth? Mom, did you go to the bathroom? Here Mom, time to take your pills."*

A huge hug, I love you, and good night.

Mom: *"Good night, Sonya. I love you."*

My turn for bed. I was asleep before my head hit the pillow.

The next day, we had breakfast with everyone and said our goodbyes. Back in the rental car to drive to Columbus then catch our plane back to Kansas City. Scott and I had our landing routine once we returned to Kansas City: After disembarking the plane, he would hop on the short blue bus to retrieve our car from economy parking. I would grab the luggage from baggage claim and wait curbside for him to pick me up. All that was the same, plus Mom.

One of the side effects of Mom's UTI and seizures the previous year, she had developed a bit of OCD about using the bathroom.

Me: *"Come on, Mom. Let's go to the bathroom before heading to baggage claim."*

March, clunk, march, clunk, march, clunk.

After retrieving our luggage, Mom and I headed curbside to wait for Scott's arrival from economy parking. The Kansas City February air was crisp, yet not completely cold. Well, for me, not for Mom. As we stood curbside, her in her long orange wool coat, she began the drill.

Mom: *"Sonya, I'm cold. It's cold. How much longer? Where is Scott?"* 1, 2, 3, 4, 5, 6, 7, 8, 9, 10...*"I'm cold."*

Dear God, give me the strength and patience to get me through two more hours with her.

Luckily, I remembered I had packed my favorite sock monkey hat on the outside of my luggage. I zipped that bad boy out and promptly put it on her head.

Mom: *"Ohhhh, Sonya. That feels warmer. Thank you very much."*

That image of her, arms folded, smiling, sock monkey hat, buttoned up in her orange wool coat is priceless. I snapped a picture. To this day, it is one of my favorite memories of her and that moment. It reminds me of her happiness and my lack of patience with her.

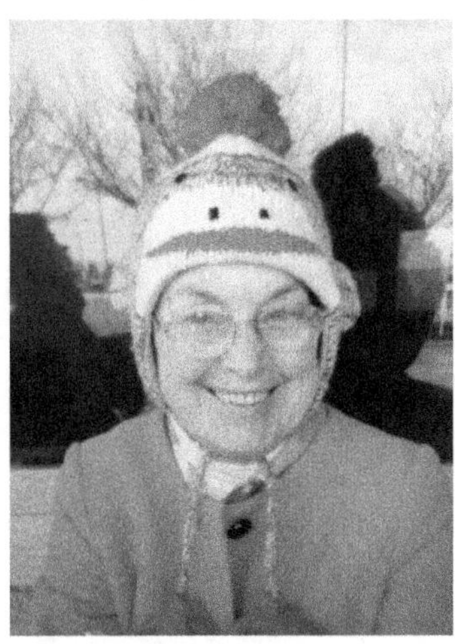

LESSON 17: Find joy. March, clunk, march, clunk, march, clunk.

16

MOTHER'S DAY

2013

One year later, our lives had settled down a bit. Scott and I returned to our daily life and work routines. Our weekends were a bit different. Our Saturday morning routine involved going to the gym, returning home to shower and dress, and then driving down to see Mom at Foxwood Springs.

Upon arriving at Foxwood, Scott and I would discuss our action plan before entering the building. We would both go to room 301 to greet Mom and say our pleasantries. Mom lit up seeing us both. Hugs all around. Then Scott would occupy Mom's attention talking about her week's activities—trips to the in-house coffee shop where the residents would sit and gossip, church activities, or that someone sat at the wrong table for lunch or dinner. While Scott was distracting Mom, I would take the garbage bag I brought and clean out her drawers and cabinets.

As Mom's dementia consumed her, her OCD-like habits grew. She developed a habit of taking Styrofoam drinking cups from the dining room located just outside her door. Her corner kitchen cabinet was jammed full of them. During my cleaning spree, I would find cranberry-colored cloth napkins that she forgot to leave in the dining room, picture frames completely disassembled (with the glass in one drawer and the picture in another), plastic touch lights completely dismantled with the batteries shoved into a drawer and hidden underneath mismatched socks, and her clothes shoved into various locations with no rhyme or reason to organization.

I was a mess as I opened each drawer. Who knew what I would find? At first, it made me mad, frustrated, and sad. I couldn't fix her; I could only try to ensure her happiness and safety.

I desperately wanted to fix her.

Mom was never officially diagnosed with OCD, yet a standing order lived on her medical chart for Ativan to calm her anxiety-based behavior. Mom's OCD took many forms as her dementia progressed. It wasn't so much OCD as it was that she would forget she had already done something. Whether it was picking up a few Styrofoam cups when she needed a drink of water, or when she couldn't figure out how to use the touch light and tried to solve it, only to take it apart, which then left it unusable.

Knowing her OCD tendencies would only grow with time, each week I would remove a few objects from her physical space to limit the clutter and chaos that existed in her mind.

LESSON 18: Your normal is not theirs.

The 245-square-foot room she lived in was efficient. The oversized door was left-hand swinging into a tiny space with the bathroom immediately to the right. The bathroom contained a toilet and shower room combination for ease of resident movement and housekeeping cleanliness. The remainder of her room was the bedroom containing her full-size bed, a dresser at the foot of the bed with a flat-screen TV, the orange boucle fabric recliner she had recovered twenty years prior (when she was still married to my father), a side table with a lamp, and the six linear feet of a corner kitchenette with brown cabinets, a sink, and under-counter refrigerator. The rectangular design was efficient and included a bay window for a touch of home. Honestly, the space delighted her; but in my mind, it was pitiful.

Every visit brought on more guilt and angst for me.

How could this be happening to her?
To me? To us? It wasn't fair.

Once the decluttering operation was complete and I had returned the napkins and pitched the cups, we would take her out for lunch. When leaving an assisted living facility, you need to sign out your loved one in the notebook and inform the nursing staff what is going on in case she needs to take her medication at lunch. The staff always encouraged Mom to have a good field trip and their eyes said to me, "Thank you for taking care of her and giving us a break."

I cannot thank all the caregivers enough for their dedication and love for Mom. While she could be the sweetest, kindest, funniest human in one moment, her anger and nastiness would come out quickly.

Mom, Scott, and I would walk down the oversized hallway, past the public restrooms and the various curio cabinets dotting the hallway. There were seating arrangements placed just so for the residents to catch their breath or rest a bit as they continued their journey. We'd walk through the glass vestibule and into the sunshine and fresh air. Deep breaths. Inhale.

There is a certain odor that exists in an assisted living facility. It smells like old age with hints of menthol from Bengay or other pain relief crème. I'm not sure if the scent lingers in the old, upholstered furniture, which might have accidentally been peed on by a resident who sat a bit too long, and when they stood up, left a bit behind. Yes, this does happen. It isn't a horrible scent, just a scent.

I wonder if a Lampe Berger could fix this?

As we walked outside, Mom would stop and fawn over the knockout roses she had planted. To her, the green shrubs with small pink roses were "her garden." I should have cared, but I didn't. To me, they were a distraction for her at the moment, a moment we should have been focused on each other. I should have cared more because they made her happy.

Me: *"Mom, doesn't the sunshine feel good?"*

She was focused on her rose bushes.
As we helped her into the car...*"Mom, where would you like to have lunch today?"*

Mom: *"A cheeseburger sounds really good, with a Coke."*
Scott: *"Deanie, that's a great idea. Let's go get a cheeseburger."*

As I rolled my eyes at my husband, I got into the car. This was our routine that played out every weekend.

Within two miles of Foxwood Springs were plenty of fast-food chains to appease Mom's cheeseburger desires. One weekend, we went to the buffet at the Golden Corral. I hated these trips because I didn't know which Mom would show up

—kind Social Mom or Angry Mom. I was always on pins and needles; I had become a helicopter parent! Small children were Mom's *shiny object*. I would give the parents a reassuring smile, which I hoped conveyed their child was safe and would be unharmed. "Please just give this lady the little joy that your child brings to her." I was terrified that one day Mom would go too far and an overzealous parent would react. Thankfully, that never happened.

At the buffet line, I helped Mom select her food. Her plate consisted of beef or chicken swimming in gravy, mashed potatoes with gravy, a roll with butter, and peas for color. Her plate was a spectrum of beige-gray food.

Me: *"Mom, would you like a salad?"*
Mom: *"No."*

I was grateful for the salad bar. The funny thing about the salad bar, it was pristine and well-stocked compared to the meat, potato, and gravy line. Not many salads are eaten in this neck of the woods. It was a small happy place for me.

Our lunch conversation was lighthearted, with Scott doing most of the talking. This was his offering. Scott's gift is that he can talk to anyone. I love this trait, and at times, I am jealous of him for it. We would share our week's events at work while walking our dog Tucker, and talk about any special architecture projects I was working on. Mom was always attentive and loved hearing about our lives. Of course, we would talk about Walt and remind her of the wonderful life they had shared. She missed him dearly. Walt was her world. On occasion, she would get misty-eyed for him and ask, *"Why did he die? What happened to him?"*

This was a story I would repeat ad nauseam. About the tenth time you tell it, you begin to leave out details so as not to overtell the story. During one Mom and daughter McDonald's lunch, Mom asked about Walt and what happened. She couldn't understand or remember the timeline that was only a few weeks old. Angry and frustrated, I pulled out my trusty notebook and drew out the Walt and Dean hospital timelines to help her remember. You can't help someone remember; they either do or don't. This was not a shining moment for me, and I remember leaving with a behemoth amount of guilt and shame for how I had treated her.

LESSON 19: They either remember or they don't. There is nothing more to it.

Typically, after lunch, we would run to either Walmart or Target to pick up a few things she needed: toothpaste, Pond's, a comb (she misplaced them), or new socks (she lost several). These were not quick trips where you run in, pick up your items, and leave. Oh no, these were excursions of walking the aisles for her entertainment. My patience was not there, but Scott's was. The last aisle was always the candy aisle to restock her dwindling supply of Werther's caramel candies. Two bags got her through the week. Dropping Mom off at Foxwood Springs was bittersweet. Yes, I loved being with her. No, I didn't want to leave her at this place. No, I couldn't have her live with us. Yes, I felt guilty.

We would escort Mom back to her room, through the glass vestibule, say hi to the rose bushes, stop to view the objects in the curio cabinet, pass the public toilet, right turn, left turn, and she was back to room 301. Scott would settle her in while I popped over to the nurses' station to officially log her back in. Responsibility baton passed back.

In her early days at Foxwood Springs, we didn't need to walk her back to her room. She knew her way. In those early days, she would sit outside the building on the black wrought iron chair, waving as we drove away. Mom gave good hugs and not a day goes by that I don't crave her hugs. She would always say, *"Thank you for taking care of me. I love you gobs and gobs."*

As we drove away, I would release a huge sigh, take Scott's hand, and say, *"Thank you for helping me. Loving her. I love you."*

Scott: *"Not a problem honey bunny. I love you too."*

17

LEGAL, FINANCES, AND SOCIAL MEDIA

2013

Getting a handle on Mom's finances was challenging. Mom and Walt had various IRAs scattered at various banks throughout the rural countryside. Still to this day, I have no clue as to why they chose to do that.

I reached out to our attorney and had him draft the proper paperwork for Mom to sign: a will and durable power of attorney (DPOA). I was the executor, with Bob being second in charge. I asked our attorney to review all the legal paperwork I had found in Mom and Walt's tiny file cabinet and lockbox. The attorney was to ensure that I had uncovered all that existed relating to any wills, titles, bonds, stocks, and insurance policies. Luckily, nothing fishy turned up, and from a legal standpoint, in the state of Missouri, Mom received all the assets.

Once the paperwork was reviewed, with DPOA in hand, and Walt's certificate of death, I was armed to start chipping away to consolidate Mom's assets into one banking account.

Wills: check.

LESSON 20: Order a minimum of ten death certificates, maybe more depending upon your circumstances. It is easier to have too many than too few.

I scheduled a trip to the local Social Security office to switch Walt's benefits to her. Mom went with me, and I can tell you, I was on pins and needles the whole time because I didn't know which Mom would show up. Thankfully, Social Mom was present that day. I asked for her checks to be electronically deposited into Mom's checking account.

Social Security: check.

Walt did have a life insurance policy we found. We also found the paperwork he had ordered to modify the beneficiaries of his life insurance policy. He never changed it, and his kids got it all. Do you know how hard it was for me to call the life insurance company, send them the information they requested, and then send Walt's kids copies of his death certificate so they could apply for the life insurance payout? Yes, I did it. And, of course, I had to do it twice because Walt's daughter Sandy lost the first one.

> *Dammit, Walt. Why didn't you take care of this?*
> *I know you wanted Dean to have this money, not them.*

Life insurance: check.

One Saturday, Mom and I took a trip to their main bank to consolidate their savings and a few IRAs into a checking account. We also added my name to the account because I would be signing all her checks and paying her bills moving forward. Mom, who had been a bookkeeper at many companies, enjoyed the trip to the bank. She was happy to be away from Foxwood for a few hours and to spend time with me.

Bank accounts: check.

While making Walt's funeral arrangements, I also took care of everything for Mom's future funeral. I had heard from other friends to use her bank funds to pay for the funeral arrangements, so you knew it was handled. Mom was to receive the same casket as Walt; she would want it that way.

Mom's future funeral: check.

Insurance coverage was a different story. Both Mom and Walt had Medicare Part B through Blue Cross Blue Shield, along with a policy from US Healthcare. Between the two policies, the majority of their healthcare bills were covered. What I needed to understand was which policy matched each of them. Once I got a handle on the insurance bills, it was a breeze moving forward. However, there was one small caveat. About a year after Walt's death, I was going through Mom's checking account, and I noticed two withdrawals for insurance. Puzzled, I called the insurance and asked why there were two withdrawals. Yours truly had forgotten to inform them that Walt had passed away! I guess I presumed they would be notified by the hospital, which didn't happen. They were completely apologetic and refunded every dime withdrawn since Walt's death back into her checking account.

Insurance: check.

LESSON 21: Make a list of all the people and companies and inform them of your loved one's death.

I am grateful Mom was not on a ton of prescriptions. All the living facilities had their partnerships with medical providers, who billed in a very timely manner. About every third Sunday morning, I would pull out all of Mom's bills and go through them. It was a routine I developed and maintained until her death. Find a rhythm and system that works for you and stick to it. I did my best to schedule autopay as much as I could, yet some companies still wanted a check.

Prescriptions: check.

I am grateful Mom and Walt were of a certain age where the internet and social media had no importance in their lives. Heck, it was a miracle they even had a flip phone! I do not have experience canceling all the various email, finance, entertainment, social media, airline, Amazon, shopping, newspaper, automatic bill pay, and the multitude of online internet accounts Mom or Walt could have created. None of this existed for them, so I didn't have to deal with this aspect of their lives. Mom and Walt had no interest in the world wide web; a good telephone land line was all they needed to connect with their circle of friends.

Yet not one to leave anyone hanging, I did a bit of research to uncover another rabbit hole of legal challenges related to canceling a loved one's accounts after they pass. Yes, the term "digital estate planning" now exists within our world, and the Terms and Conditions for each site vary along with state-by-state laws. I liked the Everplans website because it lists all the 230 plus accounts one could have, with a link to each domain and how to close the account. https://www.ever plans.com/articles/how-to-close-online-accounts-and-services-when-someone-dies [1]

Social media: nothing to do!

LESSON 22: Talk to each other! Share with your loved ones. Ask them where they keep their passwords and list of accounts. Loved ones, please share this information with someone you trust.

I am lucky that Mom's many years of working as a book-keeper and office administrator meant, for the most part, their insurance, banking, and bill pay files were in one location—the desk in the kitchen. That made it easy for me to gain a handle on which accounts to close and which I could switch over for electronic bill pay.

18

SELLING THE FARM
2013/2014

After Mom settled in at Foxwood Springs, Walt's funeral was done, my surgery was over, and Maggie's wedding was completed, our focus turned to the farm. It needed to be cleaned out and sold.

When Mom and Walt retired from the farm, they eagerly spent the weekends driving through the small towns of Missouri, antiquing. Walt collected glass oil lamps and glass cruets; Mom collected this and that. They called themselves Lucky Ducks after both having had not-so-happy previous marriages. They had a happy life of gardening, spending time with friends, antiquing, attending church, and loving life. All their goodness and fun left a house full of stuff to organize and downsize. About twenty years of belongings filled the house and basement and barns.

Starting in January of 2013, Scott and I typically spent every weekend, four-to-six hours at a time, organizing, and cleaning out the deep freezer, refrigerators, bathrooms, closets, basement, and the house in general. Who knew a frozen turkey would be in the deep freeze after three years? One weekend, we hauled over thirty large yellow trash bags to the end of the driveway for pickup. I must thank the local trash service and their staff for not asking any questions and taking every piece of garbage we left. There was an emotional limit that I could only handle every weekend. My limit—four hours at a time. I would finish one box, open another, and see utility bills from 1972 that Mom either refused to throw away or forgot. I would sit and cry, shake my head, and feel the anger of being placed in this position to deal with it. I was so sad and angry at her, at him, and at this situation.

All their clothing was donated to a local charity. Why does a grown man need fifty pairs of jeans? Some with the tags still on them.

LESSON 23: Don't leave your life for someone else to pick up the pieces.

After five months of cleaning and organizing, we brought Mom to the farm before hiring the auctioneer. On many occasions, Mom had begged to see the farm and revisit it. I had heard from several friends, that to limit your loved one's confusion, only take them back once to their former home to say their goodbyes. I am truly glad I listened. Scott and I were on pins and needles during the visit to the farm. Mom was happy to visit and be there. It had been over five months since she last stepped foot on the farm. So much life had happened to all of us. It was heart-wrenching watching her walk through her home, staring at all her possessions. I encouraged her to pick something out to take back to Foxwood. It was too much for her, she was overwhelmed with emotion and dementia fog. She was sad. I was sad. We all were sad.

Of all the things to take from the house, she selected the wooden Lucky Ducks from the bookshelf. That was all she could comprehend.

It took the auction company a week to organize everything. The sale was booked, advertised, and had the buzz of the rural country. The money raised would go into Mom's banking account to provide her with funds to pay for her new living arrangements. The auction house folks were kind and supportive of the situation; they had seen it many, many times. Their only rule: if an item was on the trailers, it could not be removed and would be sold. This was to ensure no family member would walk by, see something, and take it. Once I turned the belongings over to them, it was theirs to sell.

PANIC! I vaguely remember one Sunday, cleaning out the primary bathroom and finding an item that was shocking for a child to find because that's their parents! However, said item reinforced the avid sex life they had. Horrified, I ran to the trailer, found the auctioneer, and quietly whispered in his ear that a certain white box needed to be removed, not sold, or opened. He of course was curious, and I whispered in his ear the contents of the box (penis pump). With a wry smile, he understood. Box recovered; Walt's legacy intact. Crisis averted.

During the house emptying phase, I wish I had truly hit the pause button and walked through all the items to be auctioned to think about each piece and ensure I was ready to let it go or no longer wanted or needed it. To date, there is only one piece I wish I could have kept—Mom's orange plastic cake stand with a cover. It held many birthday cakes over the years.

The two-day auction was done, and a lifetime of treasures netted Mom $20,000. In my head, I knew that money would cover her living expenses for six months at Foxwood Springs.

Belongings sold: check.

Now to focus on painting the interior of the house and getting it on the market. A painter was hired to remove all the wallpaper, patch the walls, and paint the interior of the house to freshen it up. Lipstick on a pig. The house was ready for sale.

Thankfully, it took a few months to find the right buyer, which led to a house inspection. The old septic tank lines had collapsed which meant a new septic pond needed to be built. The south basement wall had settled a bit too much and needed steel column reinforcing. Yes, that basement wall was like that the day Mom and Walt moved in. If I wanted to sell the farm, those two items needed to be fixed.

Basement wall: check.

Septic pond: check.

Farm sold: check.

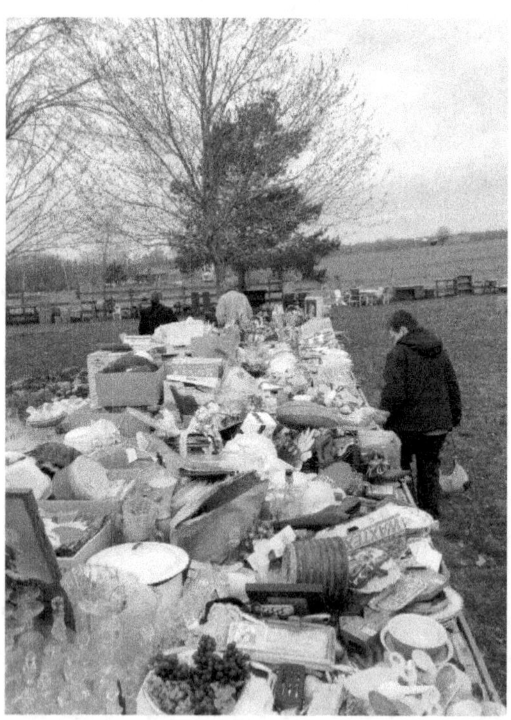

19

ACTIVITIES
2015/2016

With Mom's dementia progression, each visit it became more difficult to converse with and entertain her. I came up with what I thought was a brilliant idea, to purchase a kid's puzzle with no more than twenty large pieces and we would work on it together. As a kid, I loved puzzles. Every year in grade school during Christmas break, I would go to the coat closet and pull out every single puzzle I owned. They were of all shapes, sizes, themes, and pieces. During the break, I would commandeer the dining room table and complete all the puzzles. On occasion, Mom would join in the fun. That brown oval dining room table was my happy place working on puzzles. I had hoped bringing a puzzle to her for our visit would spark a fond memory and provide a bit of entertainment.

Oh, how I hope this works today.
Please be in a good state of mind today.

It was my typical Saturday with Mom at Foxwood Springs. I arrived a bit before 11:00 a.m. and headed to her room. That day I found her seated in the common sitting area flipping through the local Kansas City Star newspaper.

Me: *"Hi, Mom! Nice to see you!"*
Mom: *"Oh, Sonya. It is so good to see you!"*

Like a meerkat, she popped up out of the chair, dropped the newspaper, and gave me her Mom hug. You know the kind, arms wrapped tight around your body, a beaming smile on her face, both cheeks greeted with a kiss, and the inward love oozing out towards you.

Me: *"Mom, what's exciting in the newspaper?"*
Mom: *"Nothing, nothing at all."*

We chatted for a bit and moved toward a table to sit. I told her I had a surprise for her. She was intrigued. I pulled out the puzzle and said, *"Let's do a puzzle together!"* She nodded in agreement, yet with a discerning "I'm not sure" look on her face. I opened the box and dumped the pieces. We both worked to turn the pieces over with the images facing right-side up.

Me: *"Mom, let's find all the corner and edge pieces?"*

She did her best to locate the pieces, yet she struggled to identify them.
I held up an edge piece and pointed.

Me: *"Mom, we are looking for a piece that has a straight, flat edge, like this one."*

She nodded again.
Once the framework of the small rectangular puzzle was complete, it was time to infill.

Me: *"Mom, now we are looking for the middle of the puzzle. Can you find all the yellow flower pieces?"*

Again, she nodded in agreement. She began picking up random pieces even if they didn't have yellow flowers.

As I watched her pick up a piece, she would stare at it and turn it over in her hand. Her brain was trying to comprehend what it was and where it fit into the puzzle. She would take a piece and try to make it fit even if it didn't fit. Try as she might, it would not fit.

Slowly, I could feel the anger, frustration, defeat, and helplessness building up inside me.

How could this be happening?

At that moment, I remember thinking, "She is crazy and has completely lost it." I was in dementia diagnosis denial. With each piece of the puzzle, I grew more and more frustrated. I was not being empathetic to her situation, only frustrated that I was stuck dealing with this, with her.

My lack of patience got the better of me. After thirty minutes I was done. I couldn't do it anymore. We put all the pieces of the puzzle back in the box and sat. We had nonsensical conversation a bit more. In disgusted sadness, I walked her back to her room and left.

The drive home was tough. I was so sad. I was filled with so much anger and guilt. It was painful to sit and witness her inability to complete a simple kid's puzzle.

How could this be?

What was happening to her?

Dammit, this isn't fair for her

Through tears, what I was really thinking, selfishly, was that this wasn't fair to me.

Oh, poor me.

As I drove back to Kansas City, my sadness morphed into helplessness. All I wanted to do was wander and walk around with disbelief numerating through my mind. Basically, retail therapy became my crutch, and I drove to the closest shopping center to just wander. I didn't need anything except to keep moving in hopes of getting away from life's speed bump of defeat.

Oh, poor me.

During the writing of this book, my friend Mandy Shoemaker and her business partner, Michala Gibson, created Connectivities. Their vision is to create an engagement and learning tool for communities of people who may be difficult to connect with, thus, missing out on important aspects of quality of life. https://connectivities.us/

I so wish this would have been available for Mom.

20

HYGIENE

At some point in Mom's dementia journey, her interest in hygiene diminished. The habits we have developed, such as brushing our teeth in the morning and at night, we are able to remember. She did not. Even when the staff reminded her, her concentration and effort toward this task waned.

Mom grew up in the dental age of amalgam (mercury) fillings for cavities. I, too, suffered from this. For over two hundred years, dentists have used amalgam fillings and there is much debate on the health risks and side effects of having a mouthful of them. I am not here to debate this subject, yet I do believe they have negative health risks.

Due to her childhood of poor food options and lack of preventative dental care, Mom had several crowns, bridges, and fillings. Mom's mouth was filled with amalgam fillings. Before her seizures, she was fanatical about brushing her teeth and using dental floss and mouth wash to maintain her beautiful smile. Unbeknownst to me, after her seizures, she stopped brushing her teeth and bacteria took over. One day, I received the dreaded phone call from the Foxwood Springs nurse, who informed me that Mom had been complaining about a painful toothache, and she needed to see the dentist.

I arranged for her dental appointment and left work to meet her at her room and walk her around the corner to the resident Foxwood Springs dentist. Think about the situation for a moment. Who likes going to the dentist? No one I know of. I have a huge fear of dentists thanks to my childhood dentist being a toad while I was in the chair getting a tooth pulled at a young age. Imagine your own angst of the dentist, and then imagine being a human who has cognitive challenges and the inability to understand everything going on around her. Imagine the anxiety, fear, and nervousness of walking into an unfamiliar dental office, with unfamiliar surroundings, and sitting in the dental chair. I did not empathetically think about this.

The dentist was kind and reassuring, purely professional. The diagnosis: Mom needed to have a tooth pulled because it had cracked and was causing her tremendous pain. After consulting with the dentist, we both agreed that pulling the tooth was the best option. We would not put in a replacement because the trauma of an implant would be too much for her to bear.

LESSON 24: Ask the dentist for anxiety medication options to calm your loved one.

Looking back, I wish I had asked the dentist, or the doctor, to prescribe relaxation medicine for Mom to calm her nerves before pulling her tooth. Her anxiety was off the charts, yet she powered through. I sat with her in the dental room and held her hand, while reassuring her (in my best calming voice) she would be fine.

> *Dear God, please make this*
> *quick for both of us.*

The nurses would be tasked with her twice-daily saltwater

rinse to ensure a quick heal. For the next several days, I would endure repeated phone calls from her: *"Where is my tooth?" "Why did they pull my tooth?" "Sonya, I have a hole in my mouth."*

This scenario was repeated twice during the rest of her life. Between the nurses and me, we constantly reminded her to brush her teeth.

I am so sorry that you have to endure this, Mom.

When you live in an assisted living facility, you are required by state law (every location is different) to take a shower or bath twice a week. Even that was too much for Mom!

When we think of a bathroom, the memory of our own bathroom creates our baseline. We use this memory for comparison. For many reasons, some due to liability by the facility and others due to ease of cleaning by the facility, assisted living facility bathrooms are efficiently functional; not the high design you would find in *dwell, Elle Décor, or Better Homes and Gardens*. Her thirty-four-square-foot bathroom was a separate room within her bedroom. The room was tiled with 4" x 4" white tiles, with a plain-Jane (white) wall-mounted sink with a mirror above it, a wall-mounted toilet, a corner shower (complete with grab bars for safety), and a drywalled painted ceiling with a couple of dimly lit recessed can lights. The utilitarian room served a purpose. This bathroom would not win any awards; it was functional only.

The nursing staff was diligent about helping, supporting, and cajoling her to bathe. On occasion, when talking to Mom on the phone, she would complain about taking a shower.

Me: *"Mom, you need to take a shower."*
Mom: *"But, Sonya, I just had one yesterday."*

She would say that even though it had been three days. What could anyone do?

Grooming her nails was another subject. This little tidbit always puzzled me as it seemed to be part of taking care of someone. As we age, nails grow slower. Nails grow dull in color and tend to become hard and thick with ingrown toenails becoming the norm. This happened with Mom. She had developed industrial-strength fingernails and toenails. I presumed this phenomenon is the reason why the nursing staff did not want to take on this responsibility. Every month, when I knew Mom was in a good state of mind, I would trim her nails. She used to chuckle that she and Walt did this for each other.

Walt, she needs you for this! Not me.

Let's talk about hair. Mom was of the age where making a trip to the local hairdresser was a religion; you didn't miss the weekly hair appointment consisting of the wash, set, and dry that would last a week, sometimes longer. And don't forget the occasional permanent wave. Mom cherished her appointments; it was an event she looked forward to every week. During the first few years of assisted living life, she had no problem scheduling the in-house appointment and walking herself down the hallway to the Foxwood Springs beauty parlor. Yes, they still called it that.

After Mom left Foxwood and moved to Homestead, her anxiety and OCD tendencies would not allow her to sit in a chair to receive a permanent wave. She was too anxious and fidgety, and the stylists could not dedicate the time to her. One Saturday, I accompanied her to the in-house beautician to sit with her while she received a haircut. I was in awe of the beautician's patience and kindness while working on a resident.

I could learn a lot from this stylist.

She took great care with small talk to occupy Mom's thoughts and take her mind off getting her hair cut. As I sat with her, holding her hand and talking, she was as squirmy as a small child receiving their first haircut. I could sense the beautician's nervousness about potentially and inadvertently cutting my Mom. Again, I had to remind myself of her new reality and my focus on keeping her safe and healthy. Her typical hairstyle was no more.

Mom's Voicemail: 24 May 2016, at 4:47 p.m.

"Hey good evening, Sonya. This is your mother. Honey, I just wanted to speak to you and say hello and how are you doing everything. I sure miss getting to see you and everything. I love you so much So, I'm not doing anything back in the room...with...Oh...I just wish I was out of here. I hate this place...but I guess for some reason this is where I'm meant to be. You all...I love you today honey, and I always will. You're such a good person. You're a good mama, honey, Bye-bye.

PART 2

MIDDLE-STAGE ALZHEIMER'S (MODERATE)

JUNE 2015 – MARCH 2016

21

LIFE SETTLES DOWN
2015/2016

It took over a year for all of our lives to settle and formulate into a routine. My architectural job was busy, which meant I traveled every other week. Scott, too, was on the road traveling to and from Nebraska, Iowa, Missouri, and Kansas.

Normally, when my phone would vibrate or ring, I was excited to see who was calling. You know that feeling. Yet with Mom living at Foxwood Springs in Raymore, I hated my phone. I hated it when it vibrated or rang. My heart would always skip a beat when her number or the Foxwood Nurses' Station number would pop up.

I don't want to answer this.
What was happening now?

As Mom's dementia progressed, her OCD habits did as well. The telephone became her lifeline, and she would call me four-to-six times a day, sometimes more. When she moved into Foxwood, I created a simple printed phone list for her of all the people who mattered in her life that she could call. Her sisters, her church friends, her Kentucky high school friends, Bob, and me.

I learned from both Aunt Susan and Bob if I didn't pick up my phone, Mom would call them in a panic to speak to someone. If none of us picked up, she would just hang up. Of course, technology informed all of us that Mom had called two, three, four, or five times. Sometimes, she would leave a message. These messages were sad and angry. Whether she intended for the message to leave the recipient filled with guilt or not, it did. Her voice was panicky with a bit of paranoia. Someone was not treating her well. Or she would leave the voicemail begging, *"Call me, I am so lonely."*

For my sanity, I eventually had to block her phone number. Phone calls every thirty minutes during a workday were too much for me to bear. When I would have a break in the day, I would open my phone and scroll down to the blocked calls to see how many times she had called.

Four calls today, that's not bad. Sigh.

I knew she was sad.
I knew she was lonely.
I knew she missed Walt.
I knew how she felt.

I felt helpless.
I felt guilty.
I felt sad.
I felt angry.
I felt defeated.

I was mad at the situation.
I was sad knowing she was only going to get worse.
I felt empty.

As she settled into Foxwood Springs and made friends, I encouraged her to try the activities that Foxwood offered.

> **Me:** *"Please, go to church. Please, get on the bus and take the shopping trip. Please, go outside and see the blue sky and get some sun."*

She tried the bus shopping trip once and it was not a good outcome. The entire trip confused her and made her uncomfortable. I quickly learned from that one experience that she would always need someone to be with her on an excursion, and her independence was gone. The phone call I received from Mom after the bus trip was tough. She was agitated, confused, and sad.

When I would ask her if she had gone outside for the day, her response was, *"Yes, I left my room."* She didn't equate going outside to leaving the building to feel the sunshine on her face. She equated going outside to only leaving her room. I was learning a new language.

Foxwood Springs was required to call me if an incident happened. There were plenty of those phone calls:

- She had developed a habit of taking food from other people's plates without asking.
- She would get upset if someone sat in "her" chair.
- She developed a bad habit of physically lashing out at the other residents if she got upset.
- She didn't want to take the required two showers or baths a week.

Mom lived at Foxwood Springs from January 2013 through May 2015. For the first few years, she was Social Mom---happy, sweet, and easy to redirect. In early January 2015, she had grown combative, and it was not appropriate resident behavior for assisted living. There were rules, and she was pushing their boundaries. I was told to find another appropriate location for her.

While Foxwood Springs did have a more advanced dementia care wing, she did not have the finances to afford $8,000 a month. I needed to find her a more economical solution.

Remember, the decision to locate Mom near her previous home was made to encourage friends to visit her. That lasted about four months. Her friends moved on with their lives and her guest book was emptier and emptier each week. It was time to move Mom closer to us.

LESSON 25: Think deeply about where the best place is for your loved one. Where will they receive the best communal support from family and friends?

Funny how incidents or drama scenarios always happen right before a holiday weekend, isn't it? Mom's last incident (she slapped another resident) occurred a few days before Memorial Day weekend. That Friday, I spent the entire day starting at 8:00 a.m. traveling from facility to facility to find an available bed for her, this time on the Kansas side. As Mom's finances were minimal, I needed to find a facility that would accept both Medicare and Medicaid once her finances ran out.

I am extremely grateful to the many nice people I met that day. Each admissions nurse took time to ask questions to understand Mom's dementia severity and locate her in the best place. I made my way to Homestead Memory Care of Olathe—it was perfect for her.

Mom's Voicemail: 24 May 2015, at 11:33 a.m.

"Well, there's been something that has happened here in the last ten minutes, and I've got to get out of there, honey…but I don't know where I'm going to go to…So, Sonya…please…if there's any way possible that you can get down here and get me out of this place, please do. I hope you're hearing what I'm telling you, honey…I love you very much and I know you love me…Sonya, please…please help me out as much as you can, honey…I've got to get out of this place. Bye-bye."

Mom's Voicemail: 24 May 2015, at 5:47 p.m.

"Hey, good evening, Sonya. This is your mother, honey. I was just wanted to speak to you and say hello and how are you doing and everything. I sure miss getting to see you and everything, I love you so much. So, I'm…not doing anything…I'm back in the room…and oh…I just wish I was out of here. I hate this place…but I guess for some reason this is where I have to be. I love all. I love you to death, honey, and I always will. You're such a good person. You are a good mama. Thank you, honey. Bye-bye."

Mom's Voicemail: 24 May 2015, at 6:06 p.m.

"Sonya…this is…your…wa…um…daughter. I…am I…are you… too far away for me to walk up and see you? I don't know exactly where you…a…live now. Are you in the same place that you have been? Is it too far away for me to walk up there? I've just been so bored not being able to see anybody that I know and get to talk to or anything. So…that was the reason that I called you. But I do love you so much, honey, and you know that…so…I hang up now but I love ya, I love ya, I love ya."

Mom's Voicemail: 25 May 2015, at 8:04 a.m.

"Sonya, I understand you, honey...you can't jump right at me...right away...but I am so sick at my stomach. I can't...I don't feel good. I don't want nothing to eat. All I want to do is get over feeling sick...You all have a good day, honey...I love you very much...Bye-bye."

Mom's Voicemail: 25 May 2015, at 11:01 a.m.

"Sonya, this is Willa Dean calling you, honey. I'm so sorry that I had to call you. But I am so sick. I don't know what to do with myself. I don't know what to do, honey. And I know you are a distance away. So just call me back and tell me what to do. And I can figure out something or other...but I just throw up all over everything. Bye, honey. I love you. I love you and try to have a good day."

Mom's Voicemail: 25 May 2015, at 4:14 p.m.

..................18 seconds of background noise.....................

Mom's Voicemail: 25 May 2015, at 4:16 p.m.

"Ok Sonya, when you can talk...please give me a call, honey...please, please do. I miss you so much. Please, honey. I love you...Oh, I feel so terrible today...I hope, I hope you are ok...Bye-bye."

Mom's Voicemail: 25 May 2015, at 5:16 p.m.

"Sonya, I hate to bother you with this but I tell you I feel so awful. I feel so sick. I don't know what has happened but anyway, I'm going to be laying right here on the floor...probably because I don't feel like even setting up. So... I hope all of you all

are well. I hope to see you again sometime. I love you all. Bye-bye."

Mom's Voicemail: 25 May 2015, at 6:38 p.m.

"Sonya, this is Dean. I dis...I want to get out of this place where I am at here. Is there anybody there that would come and get me...get me out of here. And take me to where I need to be going. Please, honey, somebody help me out. (whimpering soft voice) Oh dear God please...dear God please get me out of here. Dear God, please come at get me. Oh, dear heavenly Father, please help me out."

Mom's Voicemail: 25 May 2015, at 6:42 p.m.

"This is Dean, you know who I am don't you? Answer me, please. Sonya, is that you that I am wanting to talk to? (whimpering soft voice) Sonya, please talk to me, honey. I feel so...oh God I feel so awful...I don't know how much longer...I can't...I think I'll die and it will all be over with."

Mom's Voicemail: 26 May 2015 2:16, at p.m.

"I understand Sonya, but I tell you I'm as sick as I have ever been in all of my life. Just standing here watching all this stuff and everything, So, anyway I just wanted to let you know that I got your message and so on. But I am sick and I'll be ok, I'll just be ok right here. I love you, honey. Bye-bye."

Mom's Voicemail: 26 May 2015, at 2:52 p.m.

". . . Sss...Sonya, you know who this is...this is your mother, honey, calling ya...I just wanted to know...what is going on? Do I have to stay here tonight? I am so sick. I can't hardly hold my head up. Everything is just making me so sick at my stomach...I can't hardly stand it. What has caused all of this? I don't understand it. So...if

you know anything better that what I have heard...please do let me know something. I love you, Sonya. Bye-bye."

Mom's Voicemail: 26 May 2015, at 4:04 p.m.

"Well, SSSonya, did you have a good afternoon, have a good afternoon, getting to see everybody and everything. That was the only reason I was calling just to see how you're doing. I love you, honey. I hope everything is going fine. Bye-bye."

22

MOM'S SECOND HOME
JUNE 2016

Homestead Memory Care of Olathe received several positive comments from staff members at competing facilities. I guess everyone is "in the know" of what's good within the long-term care facilities. In doing my research at the time, I wanted to find an age-in-place facility with welcoming staff and a Medicaid bed solution when Mom's money ran out. Homestead checked all the boxes. Sure, there were other solutions, yet Mom didn't have the funds, or they didn't have room. Fingers crossed, this would be her forever home.

Homestead Memory Care is a large building that resembles a giant house and includes a communal living area with an adjacent dining room. She would have a private room and bathroom.

She had a daily routine of breakfast, a morning activity, lunch, an afternoon activity, dinner, and bed. I continued to visit her on the weekends and take her away for lunch and a brief shopping trip. Bless her heart, when we walked into the local Target, it was overwhelming for her. Every aisle was loaded with shiny objects. Her habit of spotting a child, walking over, and touching the child increased. I got into the habit of apologizing to the parents and informing them of

Mom's dementia diagnosis. You get used to apologizing, as other people do not understand unless they have journeyed on the dementia train with a loved one. Today, when I see a daughter or son with their aging parent, I understand what they are experiencing and my heart goes out to them. Grace is good.

As time passed at Homestead and Mom's cognitive decline continued, she entered Stage 2. I gained comfort again knowing she was in a good, safe place where staff were trained to handle residents with dementia. I wanted her to be safe and happy. I knew a cure was not possible.

Time passed and our new normal became routine. And then the dreaded phone call on August 13, 2015—Mom fell and broke her left hip. I asked the nurse to send her to Research Medical Center.

Ahhh, Research Medical Center,
here we go again.

This time, the ER trip was uneventful. Doctors agreed hip replacement surgery was the right course of action, and it was scheduled a day later. Mom breezed through surgery with flying colors. Next, the challenge of her being in the hospital and healing. I had no clue how challenging Mom would be as a patient at this point in her dementia journey.

Mom was typically a happy camper. She took directions well and listened. My concern was how she would bounce back after being under anesthesia. How long would the residual anesthesia linger and affect her dementia? We all learned very quickly that Mom was a handful as her OCD took over. Ad nauseum, I informed or warned the nursing staff that Mom would pull out her IV. She would rip off her hip bandage and stand up to walk. They thought I was crazy! Little did they know.

I continued my attempts to convey to the nursing staff that

Mom was not your typical patient. Her dementia would creep in and out, and you didn't know which Dean you would get on any given day.

LESSON 26: Learn to speak healthcare.

I am sure every family tells the healthcare team about their parents' challenges. We all think we are unicorns.

What if we truly are unicorns?

My wish for the healthcare industry is to create a better intake/onboarding process for new patients with dementia. Ask better questions about the patient and their history. Develop a more informative set of questions to learn not only about the patient but about the family members involved. Below are a few of my thoughts related to my experiences that I only wish the healthcare folks would have inquired about:

- Who am I, and what is my role to the patient?
- Asked more about the patient's background. What is the patient's role within the family? Dig a bit deeper than checking the box.
- What is the patient's education level?
- Ask about the patient's behavior. Are they high-maintenance or level-headed?
- What are the loved ones' concerns with their family member staying in the hospital? (Ex: Mom ripping out her IVs.)
- Is there any background information the family member could share to make the lives of the healthcare staff easier?
- Anything the medical professionals should be made aware of?

My mantra for dialoguing with the nursing staff: Be forthcoming and tell them what you know. My expectation is for the staff to practice active listening. Most of the time they did; only a couple of instances they did not. I was very clear with the nursing staff about Mom's willpower to just get out of bed and walk, and that she would continue to remove her IV. Pain or no pain, nothing would slow her down. They shrugged it off and did not listen. The day after her hip surgery, she did exactly what I warned the nursing staff she would do. She woke up, had to go to the bathroom, removed her IVs, got out of bed, and walked to the bathroom. The staff was shocked and in disbelief. Mom's pain tolerance was over the top.

Way to go Mom! I love your tenacity!
Told you so, nursing staff.

One of the nurses, Betty, quickly recognized Mom's will and drive. We had a good chuckle about it, and she clearly understood Mom's willpower. She assured me it was under control and would not happen again. Well, it did happen again, and Mom continued to be a challenge, not only removing her IVs but picking at her hip bandage and trying to remove it. Her OCD behavior was rearing its ugly head. Around Mom's fourth day at Research Medical Center, it was time for a nursing staff change, and the new nurse, Edith, was not willing to make any concessions for Mom. She told me it was my duty to find someone to sit with Mom and watch over her.

WTF? Oh no, you won't.

I kindly reminded her that Mom was in their hospital, and it was their responsibility to keep her safe until she was ready to be released. Amazingly, they adapted with a small table and a chair stationed in the corridor outside Mom's room.

The nurses could do their duties, attend to other patients, and keep an eye on Mom.

Reminder: Be their advocate

While Mom was slow to recover, once the anesthesia wore off, she was ready to get out of the hospital and return to Homestead Memory Care Olathe. I'm not sure if she truly liked Homestead, yet she tolerated it. Maybe she *accepted it* is a better choice of words. Mom never wanted to be a burden. This characteristic inspired both Bob and me to live our lives to the fullest. She wanted us to be happy and never held us back. For me, she always reminded me of the *Little Engine That Could*. "*Chugga, chugga, Sonya. You can do it!*" she would say. She always wanted us to have more.

As Mom was recovering, I needed to find a skilled nursing bed for her once she was released. The patient advocate at Research Medical Center, Mary, was very helpful in providing a list of facilities, so I began making the calls. A couple of places did have beds for her. Yay! This was a small win, as I learned from this journey that beds are not always readily available. Facilities make money when all their beds are full; an empty bed is not good for their bottom line. I made the rounds and visited all the facilities to check them out. As my girlfriend Kathy would say, "*A place needs to have a good vibe.*" From the list, I selected Delmar Gardens, Lenexa. Why did I pick Delmar? Recently, the facility had undergone an interior renovation, and the place was clean and bright with new furniture. The nurses were helpful, kind, and welcoming, and Mom had worked at Delmar Gardens during my college days as a third job to pay for my last year of architecture school. There was something nostalgic about the place. It had a good vibe.

I let Mary know that Delmar was our choice, and whenever the hospital could release Mom, they were ready to admit her. Or so I thought. Apparently, there was one more piece of the puzzle I did not know about. I learned that once you contact a facility to relocate/move your loved one, they call the other facility's nursing staff to get the skinny on the patient. Remember all the bad habits Mom had exhibited about removing her IVs, outbursts towards the staff, picking at her hip bandage, and popping up out of bed and walking?

They do what? YIKES!

Yep, Edith, the not-so-helpful nurse told them everything negative about Mom. Mom was not the ideal recovery patient, and she made sure to tell Delmar everything.

I was pissed off.

I was not asking or wanting the nurse to lie, but couldn't she be a bit more balanced? I felt she had only told half of the story. Edith didn't consider Mom's dementia; she had expectations of typical nondementia behavior.

Dammit.

Yes, that is exactly what happened. Edith had only taken care of Mom for one shift, and she was the one who received the phone call from Delmar Gardens. Edith was more than giddy to convey to a skilled nursing facility the difficulty with Dean. I was furious! How could one person who had only worked with my Mom for one shift be the appointed person to speak as an authority on Mom's behalf? I was livid, and I am sure to this day, Edith remembers the verbal lashing I gave her. It wasn't my proudest moment, but I have no regrets.

LESSON 27: Confirm with the hospital the identity of the one person who holds the authority to speak on your loved one's behalf to other facilities and what the messaging will be.

Ensure that both of you are aligned with what can and will be shared. I am not talking about withholding any information. Just share the information that is appropriate for the new facility, so they understand all the parameters of the situation. A patient is not black and white nor are you just checking the boxes. There is a reason we call it the practice of medicine and, right now, I felt as if no one gave a damn about Mom. They were only shuffling her through the system and because she was a challenge, they wanted to get rid of her as soon as they could. Once I learned all of this had transpired, I called Mary, Mom's patient advocate, to find out what was going to happen. Mary made it right and we were able to move Mom a few days later to the skilled rehabilitation facility of Delmar Gardens, Lenexa.

Kudos to the staff at Delmar Gardens. They were wonderful at welcoming us both. As we sat on Mom's new bed, the intake nurse asked all the right questions about Mom. Medical questions: check. Drug questions: check. Legal questions: check. Food questions: check. Mom-related specifics: check. The best part of the intake session was, as we sat there, Mom became bored and stood up and walked across the room to look out the window. The nurse looked at Mom in awe; how could a seventy-five-year-old woman, recovering from hip surgery, not use a walker and just walk?

Thanks, Mom. You clearly showcased your abilities
and the person they would be taking care of.

Mom stayed at Delmar Gardens for a bit over a week. During my visits, it gave me joy to walk into the facility, head toward her room, and *not* find her there. She wasn't just sitting in her room and feeling sad. She grew stronger each day and would wander around the facility, talking to other patients and asking staff how she could help. And yet there are only so many washcloths one can fold until they lose their mind; this is what happened to Mom. She became hostile towards others, feeling helpless and alone. She needed to feel loved, wanted, and needed. She outgrew Delmar Gardens. While Mom was at Research and Delmar, Homestead Olathe kept her room. It was time to leave Delmar Gardens and return Mom home to Homestead.

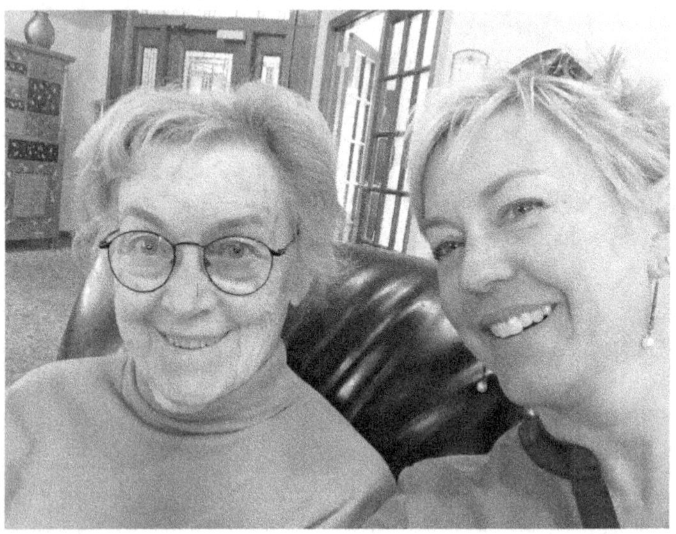

23

GERIATRIC PSYCH AND THE DREADED ONESIE

2015

Each day her short-term memory continued to fade, yet miraculously, some of her long-term memories resurfaced. She did not mention Walt's name as much; it had been three years since his passing. She also lost a lot of weight. Her size sixteen purple Gloria Vanderbilt jeans were droopy. She had gone from 165 pounds to 135 pounds. She still loved a good cheeseburger, a Coke, a small fry, and any kind of sweet, but her appetite had waned.

The communal area of Homestead consisted of open, connected spaces. After being buzzed into the front door, you signed in at the notebook and then looked around the large open family room area for your person. The room design was intended to echo the idea of someone's family room by having a vaulted ceiling, a red-brick fireplace, a too-loud TV (that was always on), and all the couches and chairs arranged in a large circle for everyone to look at each other. To me, it was pitiful to see a loved one completely hunched over in a recliner, all bundled up in a random blanket.

Was it pitiful? Was there more to be done?
My normal was not hers.

Connected to the family room, at the far end, was the large dining room with windows. The dining room had fourteen, four-foot square, brown wooden tables, and accompanying chairs typically arranged in disarray. The dining room always seemed to have a chaotic rhythm to it due to the fact the residents would move the chairs around. On one table, a puzzle of some sort would be in process with a few residents working together to complete it. At another table, you would find a group of residents chatting it up, usually with loud voices to ensure the others heard them. One or two black napkins were lying on the floor or on top of the table from where a resident stood up and walked away. Remnants of food graced the tabletops. The dining room was the heart of the facility. The residents and the staff congregated in the light-filled dining room, and there was a server window counter where you could see the hustle and bustle of the kitchen staff. More importantly, the kitchen staff could see the residents.

Every resident would greet you with a smile, and their eyes would light up seeing someone new enter their world. I had developed the habit of scanning the rooms when I entered the building to find Mom. She was my only concern, and my task at hand was to visit her in hopes of brightening her day, even if for a bit. The sad guilt was always with me.

One afternoon, I received the dreaded phone call from the Homestead nurse. We will call her Olive. Olive informed me Mom's bad OCD-like behavior of going to the bathroom anywhere had escalated, and she could no longer be trusted. She had developed a terrible habit of staying in her room, sitting in her orange recliner, and thinking it was the toilet. She would urinate in her clothes and drench the recliner. She even found the courtyard a refreshing location. This went on for a few days. They tested her for a UTI to rule it out. Nope, this was a new behavior we would need to address.

I made the purchase of adult diapers in hopes this would

rectify the situation. For about a month, it worked, and she would do her business in the diapers. But after a month, everything changed. Of course, when the nurses or I would speak to Mom about needing to use the bathroom, she would say she was fine. Then five minutes later, she would relieve herself. The challenge was she would be walking down the hallway, thinking she had to go to the bathroom, and then she would. She would pull her pants and underwear down and defecate on the floor! Mom would be horrified that I am sharing this with you, yet if I didn't, you wouldn't know how bad certain situations can be. Olive and I discussed that this behavior had been going on for about a week, and in her professional opinion, Mom needed to take a visit to the geriatric psych ward.

> *Geriatric what? What does that even mean?*
> *What happens in this place? Insert gloomy,*
> *doomy background noise from my head*
> *into your head—dum, dum, daaaaaaaaa*

I inquired what this meant, what it would entail, what she would experience, and why. Olive shared that Mom would be admitted, and the goal would be to get the medications that would be right for her. Olive thought Mom's recent change in unacceptable behavior could be due to a medical imbalance, and the doctors would slowly take her off her medications one at a time to see if that made a difference. Then they would reintroduce her medications to ensure the correct dosage. This seemed a logical approach, all things considered. It would prove not to be.

There were two geriatric psych wards within the Kansas City area, and I chose the one closest to our house—Research Psychiatric Center. Olive would make the call to the facility, and Scott and I would pick up Mom from Homestead, pack her clothes, and take her to be admitted.

I did not stop to think what this facility would look like, either internally or externally. I did not stop to think what would happen to her once she was inside. I did not stop to think about any of this.

God, please forgive me for
putting Mom through this.

We arrived at the Research Psychiatric Center. I did my best to explain to Mom that she needed to visit a different facility for a few days to help with her bathroom issues. With me, Mom was compliant and would go along with what I told her. She would look at me and say, *"Ok, if you think this is for the best."*

Guilt, guilt, guilt.

We escorted her into the building. A large waiting room with shades of faded blue and beige filled the space, with rows of waiting chairs. Mom and Scott settled into a couple of chairs, and I walked over to the reception window. I felt like I was walking up to a police station window where the on-duty officer was perched behind thick bulletproof glass. I gave the receptionist Mom's ID and insurance cards to get her checked in. The place was dreadful, and it started to hit me—I was leaving my mother here. The anxiety, the angst, and the sadness was overwhelming.

WTF?

I was so grateful Scott ran interference with Mom. He had a knack for making her smile and laugh. It gave me comfort to watch the two of them together.

I am so lucky he loves her and me.

I sat down and joined them. While it seemed like an eternity for them to call our names, I was happy for the time but scared shitless for what we all were about to experience. The receptionist called her name, and we escorted Mom through a locked door (where we had to be buzzed in), through another beige hallway with nasty, dingy fluorescent lighting, and toward the admissions office.

All three of us sat down across the desk from the admissions nurse. Her office was septically sterile and uninviting; this was not meant to be an inviting place. She had her process of asking questions and typing into the computer the details of Mom's recent events. The admissions nurse was nice enough, yet focused on the procedure of getting this new patient checked in. I asked questions about what would happen to her. What was the procedure? The nurse gave political answers, just enough to answer the question but not enough to give me a full picture. And lastly, I could only visit Mom for one hour a week on Saturday.

WTF? Are you kidding me?

I hugged Mom, kissed her, and told her I loved her. Scott did the same. Mom looked at us both with trust and sadness. I knew she knew what was going on. We walked out of that godforsaken facility, and I just cried. I bawled my eyes out. I couldn't believe I had just left my Mom at this horrible, nasty, ugly facility. I was a horrible, horrible daughter. How could I do this to her? We sat in the parking lot and cried together. The car ride home was the quietest, saddest ride ever. For the rest of the day, I felt like I was in a surreal out-of-body dream and floating through time. I couldn't get the memory of her or that place out of my mind. My whole body ached with sadness. Scott did his best to coach and cheer me up. My heart ached.

> *You are doing the right thing.*
> *Even if this is hard, it is the right thing.*

Saturday rolled around, and it was time to visit Mom. My heart ached to see her. How was she doing? Had any of this worked? Would she be ready to be released? Neither the staff nor the doctors were communicative.

We arrived, checked in at the waiting room reception desk, and waited for our escort. The escort arrived and buzzed us through the locked waiting room door into the beige hallway. We walked toward another set of double doors, the escort entered the code, and we walked into Mom's unit. Pale blue walls greeted us, and there were the nasty fluorescent lights again. Eerily, scenes from *The Shining* popped into my head. As we walked toward the center of the unit's nursing station, I saw a shape from behind, slumped over in a wheelchair. As we got closer, the escort pointed to the figure. This was Mom!

My heart sank to my stomach. Mom was in a navy blue sweatshirt and sweatpants, her head was tilted to the side, her eyes were glazed over, and she was drooling. I bent over to hug her. All I wanted to do was hold her and make it all better. She didn't recognize either of us. I looked at Scott with horror. This was not my Mom. She didn't deserve this.

> *What had they done to her? Why?*

My sadness immediately turned to outright anger and disdain. This was unacceptable, and I wanted to speak to a doctor. This was not what I had expected. We asked the nurse to locate a doctor. He did and escorted us into a small blue conference room where we waited for the doctor.

The doctor arrived and proceeded to mansplain her condition and situation. Of course, I was vocal and shared that her current state was unacceptable and that medicating her to a drooling human was not right. The doctor would not speak to me; he addressed Scott. During the conversation, Scott politely told the doctor to speak to me. *"Dean is her mother, not mine."* The doctor continued his explanation to me about dementia and Alzheimer's and that this was the procedure for someone like Mom. I was livid with his condescending attitude and lack of true concern or care for Mom. She was an object, not a human, and his approach was very clinical. All I wanted was her release.

Blah, blah, blah, doctor.

Mom stayed at Research Psychiatric another week, and they finally released her. For me, it was a joyous, happy day of freeing her. We picked her up and headed to McDonald's for a cheeseburger, a small fry, and a Coke. After lunch, we drove her back to Homestead. Ahh, safe and sound for her, for me, for all of us. To this day, I still do not know what they did to her—if her medications changed, or if it was a total ruse from Homestead to get her out of their building for a bit.

When we checked Mom back into Homestead, it came with a caveat to manage her OCD-like bathroom behavior. Enter the adult onesie. Believe it or not, an adult onesie exists. It is a jumpsuit with a zipper placed on the backside so the individual cannot pull down their pants and use the bathroom anywhere. They do exist, and I found them online and purchased three for Mom.

Let's talk about the dreaded onesie or the *Alzheimer's Special Needs Clothing One Piece Jumpsuit.* Google it. They make them for both sexes in all shapes and sizes. These are sad, ugly uniforms, yet they serve a purpose, which I never knew existed. Some loved ones can develop the habit of disrobing in public. Think of the movie scene in *Friends with Benefits,* when the dad takes off his pants before eating lunch in a public place, and the son, Justin Timberlake, follows suit to support his father. Cute scene and appropriate. In Mom's case, the *Alzheimer's Special Needs Clothing One Piece Jumpsuit* kept her from defecating in public and would give the Homestead caregivers relief from cleaning up after Mom. Mom had become a higher maintenance resident, and this was not heading down a rainbow-laden path.

The onesie worked for a bit, but Mom was still not back to a certain sense of normalcy. Olive called again and gave me the update that Mom's agitation and nervousness had become too much for the staff to handle. Essentially, Mom was unpredictable and needed someone to keep an eye on her. Homestead did not have the resources for this, and Mom needed another trip to a geriatric psych facility to make her a bit more compliant. I pleaded with Olive, *"Was there another way?"* I couldn't send her back to that place. It was horrible, and they didn't treat her well. Olive said the Saint John Hospital's Senior Behavioral Health Center in Lansing, Kansas, would be much better. They had sent several patients to this facility with success. Reluctantly, I said yes.

I picked Mom up the next day, and we made the sixty-minute drive to Lansing to check her in. The Behavioral Health Center was cleaner and nicer than the former psych facility. Also, they were in the process of updating the unit where Mom would stay. The entire process of admitting Mom was completely different and a much better experience. The staff cared, and it showed by the way we were greeted and escorted through the process. I was hopeful this would work. Mom stayed at the facility for a week, and it worked. She was calmer, less agitated, and not drooling!

When I received the call from the Behavior Health Center, the nurse, Susan, said Mom was ready to be released and could return to Homestead. I called Olive at Homestead to inform her I would be picking Mom up in a few days and would move her back to Homestead. In not so many words, Olive said no. Olive informed me that Mom had reached a point in her dementia that made her unfit for Homestead. Olive never said it, but I know Mom's agitation, defecation in public, and unruliness were too much. They didn't want to deal with her. By law, or Homestead's risk management policy, Olive could not say that, and she danced around the issue. I would need to find another place for Mom.

I called Susan back at the Behavior Health Center to inform her I needed a bit more time, as I would need to find Mom a new home. Thank goodness for Nurse Susan. She shared with me that they had trouble with Homestead not taking residents back after a stay with them. She also informed me that, per the State of Kansas healthcare regulations, they could not do this. They legally had to take Mom back, and she mentioned I could call the State and report Homestead to them. I happily called the State.

I called Olive back and informed her Mom would be returning to Homestead in a few days, and that I had called the State of Kansas and lodged a formal complaint. Olive said they would be happy to take Mom back, and they did.

LESSON 28: Know their rights. Each state is different.

I moved Mom back to Homestead for a bit, and I began my search to find her a new home. I knew it was a matter of time before Mom would lash out at another resident or do something else that would get her expelled from Homestead. My first call was to one of the places I wanted for her a few years before—Garden Terrace at Overland Park.

LESSON 29: As I mentioned earlier, there are many types of facilities, for all the various types of long-term care, prevalent in our world. Find the one that is right for your loved one and their situation.

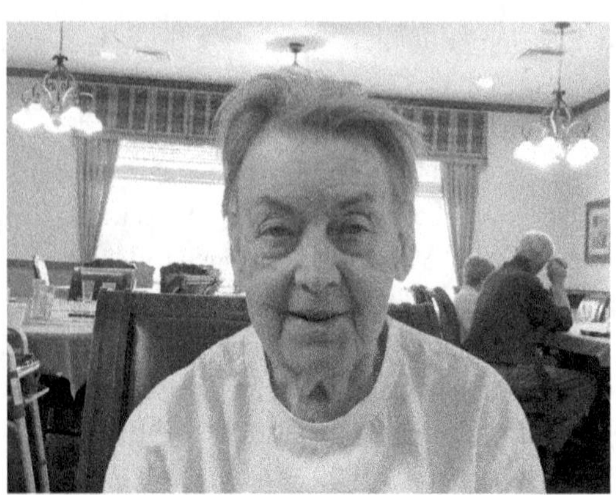

PART 3

LATE-STAGE ALZHEIMER'S (SEVERE)

MARCH 2016 – APRIL 2017

24

———————

ANOTHER PHONE CALL
MARCH 2016

After Mom's trips to geriatric psych, her dementia progressed quickly. I don't know how else to describe it: she was sad, her spunk had diminished, her physical body was shrinking in front of my eyes, and the light in her beautiful green eyes was a little less bright. I am thankful she always recognized me and Scott. She continued to light up with her beautiful smile when she saw us. And if she could, she would eagerly stand from her chair to hug us—a solid full-body Mom hug. Her ability to communicate and formulate coherent sentences was strained. Mainly, her responses were yes or no or by shaking her head. She was eating less, napping more, and seemed to be in an in-between stage of dementia. While not quite all of her cognitive skills were gone, she would still have days of normalcy. She had moved toward Stage 3; I see that now.

Early March 2016, I received another phone call from the nurse at Homestead Memory Care. Mom was complaining of pain in her right hip.

From this point, I will allow my postings from Mom's Caring Bridge website to continue this story.

LESSON 30: I set up a CaringBridge website. I should have done it sooner.

The Journey Continues: 9 March 2016

Hi, All.

This is Sonya, and I have thought on many occasions to start a CaringBridge site for Mom. It would allow me to share her journey from dementia to Alzheimer's while allowing each of you to send thoughts and prayers to her. Today is the first day of the new site. I expect to post when a significant event happens.

Yesterday, a significant event happened. I received a call from Homestead Memory Care in Olathe from Amanda Lopez, the director of the facility. On Sunday 6 March 2016, Mom was complaining of pain in her right hip/leg and was having difficulty putting any weight on it. No one witnessed a fall, so they were unsure as to why she was having pain. She stayed in bed for a couple of days, then on Tuesday it had reached a point to take the next steps and get an X-ray. We waited for a mobile X-ray, but after three hours of a no-show, it was time to move to Plan B—an ER visit.

We took her to Shawnee Mission Medical Center. After the X-ray and a CAT scan, it was confirmed there was a slight fracture in her right hip. Currently, we are waiting to see the orthopedic surgeon, Dr. Smith, to determine when surgery will occur. She is not in pain and snoring away in bed!

Comments:

"Wow, mom on the net! Who'd a thunk it? Rest easy mother…"
   —Bob Likins, 14 March 2016

Avulsion Fracture: 9 March 2016

Before today, I had not heard of an avulsion fracture; now it has been added to my lexicon. I met with Dr. Todd Smith, an orthopedic surgeon, this afternoon and he confirmed the diagnosis. Surgery is not an option because of its location and because typically these fractions heal on their own with time. Any pain will be managed with medication but not a concern at this time. Mom has slept 80 percent of the day. She did fairly well with lunch but kept spitting out her meds. The nice PT/OT ladies just left—Leslie/OT and Laura/PT. Mom took a walk, twenty feet total; she needed lots of help. If she could stay focused on walking, she could do it. Alas, the conundrum of dementia and all the "shiny objects" she sees distract her. Mom will be in the hospital until we can find her a skilled nursing facility (SNF) that can take care of her. Dr. Smith has given orders for her to walk, as she can use a walker, with no restrictions. If only she would remember to use the walker! She is resting peacefully now after thirty minutes of activity; poor gal is exhausted!

We wait to see how she does over the next few days and hope (fingers crossed) that a spot at Garden Terrace is available for her.

It's amazing the number of folks we have spoken with in a matter of twenty-four hours:

- Dr. Todd Smith–Ortho
- Beth–Dr. Smith's assistant
- Susan–Nurse of the day
- Mason–Technician
- Laura/Leslie–PT/OT
- Dr. Stephanie Million–Attending assistant
- Dr. Becky Messliri–ER Doc
- Dr. Nelpher Hathiary–she met Mom in the ER yesterday

- Keith–Pharmacist from yesterday
- Jason–ER nurse
- Glenda–Housekeeping
- Louis Perrigo–Chaplain

That's sort of an insane number of folks for *one* patient!

Garden Terrace: 11 March 2016

Mom was released by the hospital yesterday, and we moved her to the skilled nursing facility of Garden Terrace. I tried to relocate her to Garden Terrace after her hip surgery last fall, but there were no available beds. Yesterday, there was a bed! She is doing fine and walking, just sleepy. She is not in any pain.

If you would like to drop her a card, her mailing address is:

Willa Dean Mitchell
Garden Terrace of Overland Park
7541 Switzer Road–Bed A2303
Overland Park, Kansas 66214

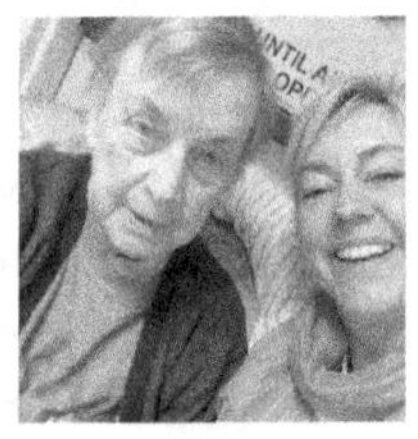

You might be asking yourself, "Will she return to Homestead?" No. While Homestead was a good place at a certain point in time, her progression requires a bit more help and a caring eye. Mom will remain at Garden Terrace for the rest of her life. While that sentence might seem harsh, is it the reality? Garden Terrace has everything she will need to ensure her quality of life and her health is good. They have an on-site doctor, dentist, podiatrist, a robust physical therapy department, and lots of engaging activities for their residents. The staff is great. This will be a good home-sweet-home for her.

Comments:

"Just got your note today and checked out the site. Wow! Sounds like it has been a bumpy road! Glad Mom is resting comfortably and is in a good place. But let's be honest...getting old really stinks! Hugs to all!"
   —Raelene Herdon, 16 March 2016

"Bless her heart, she's quite the trooper...you both are. Hugs, C"
   —Cathy Jury, 18 March 2016

**Forty-eight-Hour Meeting and Sunday Visit:
14/20 March 2016**

Garden Terrace schedules a forty-eight-hour meeting with all the directors to understand, listen, and learn more about a resident. Our meeting was on Monday, 14 March. We met with the directors of Nursing, Physical Therapy, Occupational Therapy, and Social Worker. Thank goodness I had prepared a written document about Mom and her history from the last four years of assisted living. The staff was uber pleased to have such a succinct wealth of knowledge about Mom, both personal and medical-oriented. I am pleased with her new home and the staff for asking all the right questions.

When I went upstairs to visit Mom, she was up and seated on the love seat staring at the ground. The TV was on in the corner, but she had no interest. I tried to walk with her, again with no interest.

Yesterday, Scott and I popped by to visit with her. She was

trying to get out of the recliner but was having issues pushing herself up and out of the chair without significant help. The nurse helped her up and promptly relocated her to the adjacent recliner. She had a drink of water and an oatmeal cookie, then she went back to sleep.

You may have noticed in these postings that I haven't discussed phone calls. You see, Mom can speak but her sentences are gibberish and make no sense. It breaks my heart to type this, but I want to share with each of you the brutal reality of this wicked disease. Both Scott and I have learned to speak gibberish with her, and it makes her laugh. I can't ask for anymore.

Keep your positive thoughts and prayers headed our way.

Peace,
Sonya

Comments:

"Poor mom... ☹"
  —*Bob Likins, 21 March 2016*

"So glad to hear from Dean. Wish I could communicate with her. Thanks for informing me about CaringBridge."
  —*Juanita Porter, 21 March 2016*

Just another Sunday: 3 April 2016

I visited with Mom today and found her snuggled in bed snoozing. I spoke with Ariel, the nurse of the day, to understand her activities. She had finished lunch, needed to use the bathroom, and then asked to take a nap. Ariel shared that Mom is doing fine and occasionally her aggressions show up. For the most part, she is easily directed.

On Easter, I visited and was shocked to find Mom's left

eye bloodshot! The staff had no idea what happened.

Today, her eye was back to normal and healed itself.

Mom's hip isn't bothering her as it continues to heal from the avulsion fracture.

Today, Mom asked if I was going to crawl in bed with her and nap. I chuckled and said, *"Another day."* She also asked if it was okay to go to heaven. With a tear in my eye, I said, *"Yes, Mom. That would be just fine."*

Comments:

"Thanks for visiting her, Sonya!"
  —Bob Likins, 3 April 2016

"Hi, Sonya. I am the daughter of Arlen and Betty Mitchell, and I read all of your posts to them. They were very close to your Mom and Walter. I will read this to them tomorrow, as it is late today. I know they, too, will have a tear in their eyes. Blessings to you and your sweet mama!!"
  —Susie Gray, 3 April 2016

"Makes me so sad. But I'm glad to hear from her. Thanks to you, Sonya!"
  —Juanita Porter, 4 April 2016

"Thanks, Sonya, for your updates! I read them all to my mom. She is always asking me if there are any new updates on your Mom. I know these are tough times for you and tough to make the right decisions for your Mom's care. Your Mom always bragged on you! Our thoughts and prayers are with you."
  —Karen Yoakum, 13 April 2016

"Visited Dean's site today and read all the posts. This is a very good way to keep abreast of her condition. Thanks, Sonya, for setting this up for everybody. Sharon and I will keep praying for her. It may be that question, 'Is it ok to go to heaven?' was an implied request for you to release her because she is getting tired of fighting the disease. Just a thought. Ha!"
    —*Harroll Mitchell, 24 April 2016*

UTI's...Oh My!: May 2016

It's official, Mom has another UTI (urinary tract infection). For those who don't know, UTIs are a VERY common part of the aging process and can wreak havoc on a person. Mom seems to get them twice a year. The UTI tends to make her grumpy and not quite herself. Nothing that can't be fixed with simple medication. She doesn't drink much water these days, even if you ask her! Thus, a UTI will happen.

Other than that, she is her happy, sleepy self.

Comments:

"So sorry for another "roadblock." UTI is no fun. Tell her I am thinking about her.
    —*Juanita Porter, 4 May 2016*

"Sending love from the Mitchells and Grays in Pleasant Hill."
    —*Susie Gray, 5 May 2016*

"She's not drinking because they're not feeding her some fried okra!!! Heal up quickly, mom!"
    —*Bob Likins, 5 May 2016*

"How is Willa Dean doing? Yoakum's checking in on everyone."
 —*Karen Yoakum, 22 June 2016*

25

ANOTHER DECISION
APRIL 2017

The previous year was uneventful for Mom, who had settled into living at Garden Terrace. She slowly recovered from the avulsion fracture and day-by-day grew mobile so she could wander her unit. Eventually, we moved Mom upstairs to a secure unit where I needed to punch in a code to visit her. This ensured her safety and her loved one's peace of mind. Scott and I would visit her on Saturdays, but rarely at this point did we take her away from the facility. I'm not sure if it was too much for me or her; we chose to bring her a cheese-burger, a Coke, and fries. Yes, her eyes still lit up when we visited with food. Scott was great at making small talk and making her laugh. I don't know what it was about this last stage. I knew at some point she was not longing for this world, and secretly I said a little prayer each night for her to crossover. It was gut-wrenching seeing her in this state of being. I knew she didn't want this for herself, as she had witnessed her own mother and a sibling in this state of being.

Dear God, please take her.
She doesn't want this.
Please take her to visit Walter.

On Tuesday, 18 April, the Garden Terrace nurse called to inform me that Mom fell three different times over the past ten days. The X-ray revealed an impacted fracture in her left hip, toward the very upper tip of her hip bone. According to the nursing staff and doctor, she was not in any pain, thank goodness.

But do we operate? Can we operate?

Her right hip replacement surgery was in 2015, and she was more alert and stable then. She was pretty close to being Normal Mom.

Can she even handle another surgery?

In this moment, she has no appetite with limited ability to chew and swallow completely.

What to do?

I stumbled upon a no-nonsense article regarding end-of-life care. The question the physician asked the family in the article was, *"What would your Mother's wishes be?"* A simple question that resonates down to your soul; It was a question I pondered over and over. The answer was simple. She would not want this quality of life. She would want to go to heaven. My heart, soul, and mind were all in agreement—it was time to let her go and ask the doctor for palliative care. I called my brother that night to share the sad news.

Wednesday 19 April

I met with Dr. Hodges to discuss her hip, surgery, and the next steps. I am eternally grateful for the candid and compassionate conversation with Dr. Hodges. He has been at Garden

Terrace for many years and witnessed residents come and go. The day before, he shared with me that because of the location of the hip fracture, surgery was not an option. I shared with him my angst and conversation with my brother; we were both aligned. My eyes welled as I spoke the words, *"Mom wouldn't want this quality of life, it's time for hospice."* Surreal words were uttered, and I felt the proverbial weight lifted.

> ***Am I a horrible daughter? No.***
> ***Mom wouldn't want to be a burden.***
> ***She would support our decision.***

Dr. Hodges explained that Mom would be placed into their hospice program, Comfort Care. Honestly, I was so tired and numb at that point, I was like a small child agreeing to everything he said to me. I guess I was in shock. Dr. Hodges walked with me up to Mom's unit, pulled out her chart and wrote the orders into it. To my surprise—Lacey is here today! Wahoo! Lacey has been a constant in Mom's life since she moved into Garden Terrace on March 11, 2016. Caregiving is stressful, and Lacey had recently shifted and was no longer the head nurse for Mom's unit—the English Ivy wing. Between us girls, she doesn't make enough money for the daily stress. This has been a constant theme in Mom's healthcare journey with caregivers.

Within minutes, the nursing staff, caregivers, and those who needed to know received the news. You could feel the news roll through the building from top to bottom. Of course, it is a natural human response to feel sadness once the decision is made, but I give credit to the staff for the hugs and acceptance. Comfort Care discontinued all medication except for pain (generic morphine) and Ativan to calm anxiety.

I gave it one last effort, and I tried to feed Mom lunch. She had no interest.

For dinner, the staff sat her at a table with food. When I walked into the unit, I found her hunched over, slumped is a better word, with a plate of food in front of her. Another bridge to cross and direct staff to stop shoving food in her mouth. I later learned in the State of Kansas, regulations require staff to "force" food into a resident. Here's where dementia and regulations/politics do not mix. A natural path of aging is for a human to lose interest in food. We have a built-in mechanism telling our bodies we have reached the end of the journey. We only need to listen. While the conscious living has a hard time respecting this, as we do not wish our loved one to move on, we need to listen. There is no greater love than to respect another's wish for end-of-life care.

Tonight is bath night, and I leave Mom in good hands. Once home, I fire up the laptop and write the following to place in her chart the next day.

Dear Garden Terrace Caregiver –   *19 April 2017*

To respect Willa Dean's wishes, we have asked for Comfort Care. We desire our mother to be comfortable, pain free and peaceful.

-   *If she is sleeping during mealtimes, please do not wake her.*
-   *Do not presume she is hungry. Ask her if she is hungry first.*
-   *There is to be no nudging/coaxing her to eat or drink. Meaning, do not put food on a spoon and stick it in front of her mouth.*

Thank you for all you do for our Mother!
God Bless
The Family of Willa Dean Mitchell

26

GARDEN TERRACE DIARY
APRIL 2017

To this day, I have no idea why I chose to capture the final days of Mom's time on earth. I am glad I did. At the time I searched and searched for articles, books, and stories to explain to me what happens to the human body when someone is dying. I am leaving them unedited as I want the reader to experience my stream of consciousness.

Thursday 20 April: Breakfast

With guilt, I arrive at Garden Terrace knowing I only have breakfast time for Mom today. I try to feed her, but she has no interest. I respect her wishes, somehow her body knows. She knows me today.

Friday 21 April: Lunch

Today the residents of the English Ivy wing are restless. It's like watching the YouTube video where people are recording baby pandas at Christmas time! It is a thing, Google it.

I find Mom hunched in a wheelchair with her head back

on a makeshift pillow. If this is Comfort Care treatment, then we need to change the method of care! She has those stupid blue elephant pillows strapped to her feet for protection. The irony is the Velcro on the pillows doesn't work, and they provide no protection. I quickly remove them, toss them aside, and tell the nurse how disgusting they are. Her comment: *"They wash them."*

Yeah, whatever.

The nurse pops over and asks if I am going to feed her, I'll give it a try. Diana is on staff again today. She shares that she fed Mom a cookie. I give Mom a bit of water. Immediately, said cookie and water projectile out of her mouth onto her shirt. Yep, she's not interested in swallowing.

Mom recognizes me today and smiles with "I love you." I wait till lunch is over and ask the staff to move Mom into her recliner for better comfort and sleeping. Once she is tucked in, I leave.

Saturday 22 April: Lunch

I arrive at lunch to find Mom soundly sleeping in her bed. She is tucked in, and I do not wake her. I just give her a gentle, loving caress on the head. Diane greets me with a huge hug and empathetic support. She asks if I want to feed her. I say, "Let's let her sleep."

I turn on Pandora to the Johnny Cash station and place my phone on her pillow. Mom loved Johnny Cash, and the station plays the old country western songs she loves. Somehow, I hope she subliminally hears the music. "Daddy Sang Bass" is playing—her favorite. Tears well in my eyes.

Sleep. She jerks and wakes herself up for thirty seconds of gibberish hallucinations. I tell her I love her, hold her hand, and caress her arm. Mom's right eye doesn't want to open all the way. There's brief movement and then she's back to sleep. Sadness, helplessness, and a broken heart rip through me.

One of the ladies living in the English Ivy wing is Effie. I met her grandson Matt yesterday. Nice young man with her eyes and smile. Effie used to work at the Nelson Atkins Museum as a secretary back in the day. I am so pleased to know her history and to think about who she met. She is a spunky lady with style and grace. We've had a good few days together, walking the long corridor, holding her hand for support. Two caregivers bring Marsha, Mom's roommate, into bed. This poor lady needs two people to assist her every day to and from her bed, to the table, back to bed, to a recliner, to the bathroom, and then it starts all over again. Why do we do this? The quality of life for this lady is senseless. Marsha is a giggler, which makes me chuckle.

Another resident, Sadie, is married to Frank. They moved to Kansas City from Erie, Pennsylvania. And now Frank visits Sadie every day for lunch and dinner to feed her. I witness his frustration when she doesn't want to eat and gives him an emphatic "NO!" He is a kind, loving, patient man. You can see the loving sadness on his face as he urges Sadie to eat. This is a scenario played out daily. At what point is it enough? He is not ready to let her go.

In the afternoon, the nurse loaded up a syringe and pushed liquid morphine into Mom's mouth.

Timmie and Laura assist Mom to the restroom. Mom urinates a bit which is kind of a surprise since she has not been drinking. Once the ladies return her to bed and tuck Mom in, she says, *"I love you, Sonya, and I am sorry."* I whisper in her ear, *"Mom, I love you, and I give you permission to go to heaven."* She responds with, *"I love you, Sonya."* I kiss her forehead as she falls asleep.

Oh, my heart.

Sunday 23 April: Lunch

I arrive around 11:30 a.m. to a sleeping Willa Dean. Bless her heart, all the mouth breathing has given her a horrendous case of halitosis. Poor thing, it's part of the aging process. I tell her I love her and ask, *"Are you ready to go to heaven?"* Her answer, an emphatic, *"Yes!"*

At 12:25 p.m., Pandora is on the Johnny Cash station, Mom sleeps with Willie Nelson's "City of New Orleans" playing in the background.

I remembered I had a bunch of Mardi Gras beads, and I brought them today. I passed out pink Mardi Gras beads to all the ladies of English Ivy. What a hoot to see them smile! It warmed my heart. The staff rounds up the ladies for lunch and the process of wheeling everyone into the multipurpose room to their dedicated spot begins. It wreaks havoc with the ladies if they are not at "their" spot.

I woke Mom to ask her if she was hungry.

Me: *"Mom, are you hungry?"*
Mom: *"No, I am not."*

Mom falls back to sleep, and I sit in the brown recliner. I asked the nurse for a different bed for Mom, one of the ICU beds that has a billowed mattress with air to limit any sore spots on her body. Even though she only weighs 100 pounds, she will get bed sores, and we do not want that. I also ask the staff not to cut her hair anymore.

Monday 24 April: Lunch

The pandas are restless today! Mercy, all the commotion.

Timmie shares that Mom was anxious this morning, and they gave her medicine to calm her down.

No lunch today. She had maybe one-half cup of

water/grape juice. She has been in and out of reality, complete with gibberish. There's been lots of talk about puking, peeing, and pooping. Mom's best comment today was, *"Charles didn't drink alcohol."*

Her hand strength is amazing for someone who hasn't had food for six days. Her body temperature is elevated today for the first time. This is a sign.

Today, I put my hand on Mom's chest to feel her heartbeat. It is strong and regular. I waved my hand half an inch in front of her eyes, no blinking or response. I brushed her hair and cleaned her face and applied a bit of moisturizer. I also swabbed her mouth.

It's 5:12 p.m. and the drugs have kicked in and she is snoozing, this time with her mouth closed.

Tuesday 25 April: Morning

It's interesting witnessing the unit wake up.

These staff members are so focused on the safety of the residents, but the design of the unit doesn't allow for 100 percent safety. Design could fix this and make the unit better. Yet I know this is a 1970s facility; healthcare is different today.

Design note: All the closet doors in the resident rooms need to be fitted with lights, so when doors open, lights in the closets come on. It would make the staff's job easier to select clothes and dress residents, and then the staff can move on to the next one.

Peacefully sleeping, Mom undid her brief and scratched at a spot on her nose, which led to blood on her face. I need to trim her fingernails as she is a picker. Mom continues to pull covers over her head. I place a blanket over her head with just her face peeking out—problem solved. Maybe she needed more comfort? Her body temperature is elevated again.

Staff note: Is the staff trained to deflect and tell little white lies? I've witnessed too many times staff trying to convince people and have a valid discussion.

Jennifer, the nutrition gal, stopped by and we went through Mom's orders for nutrition. Discontinue everything including nutritional drinks. I am shocked by the number of times I have had to tell the nurses/staff to stop feeding her. Each time I do, I feel like I am doing the wrong thing, even though I know it is her wish.

Today is weight day on the English Ivy unit; mercy, what a process.

Bath day for Mom is in the evening.

Scott returned home from Denver.

Wednesday 26 April: Morning

I met Effie's son Matt today while visiting her. I accompanied Effie on a walk; she was sad and crying today. Effie is ninety-four! OMG! She is amazing for ninety-four, bless her heart. Yesterday, when I accompanied Effie on a walk, she told me I was sweet. We walked down the Hibiscus Lane wing and back and she kept walking even more.

Today, I made this real by sharing Mom's story with Mom's high school girlfriends, Verna Jean and Juanita. I also shared it with our friends Donna, Kathy, the Johnsons, David, and Neal. No matter how many times I share the story, it doesn't get any easier.

Mom is solidly sleeping. Bless her heart.

I dashed out to lunch with Scott to Thai Orchid. Man, oh man, spicy Pad Thai! Mercy, my mouth was on fire.

Today was a cold and misty day in Kansas City. I left Garden Terrace around 5:00 p.m. to go home and eat dinner at Nara. Yum.

Mom's breathing is interesting. She reminds me of a goldfish out of water with mini gasps of air. She continues to bend her right leg and rub her shin and foot.

Thursday 27 April

Yoga morning for me; I needed that.

Mom was awake and a bit agitated, so I asked for the Roxanal to calm her and me. She is restless and moving her legs quite a bit today. Within twenty minutes, the Roxanal takes over.

I met Harriet—quiet, smiling Harriet.

I had lunch with Kathy and Scott at Dos Reales; I am so grateful for my friends.

A song by Pink Floyd played in my mind, describing how I felt—comfortably numb. Thank you, Pink Floyd, for the lyrics.

The English Ivy unit is extremely noisy today. Marjorie (a very vocal resident) wouldn't shut up.

I have a work event in the evening/afternoon at University Health and then dinner at home with Scott.

Friday 28 April

I spoke with Amanda about the whole Comfort Care gig. They are not turning Mom every two or four hours. She was awake and agitated when I arrived at 9:30 a.m. There was a sound machine going—a heartbeat. WTF? Gotta fix this.

Effie isn't her normal spunky self; they modified her medication. Poor lady.

My heart is so heavy today, and I can feel the emotional weight on my shoulders.

Mom has pinpoint pupils and continues to sleep.

Her roommate Marsha is in bed after lunch, talking to herself and giggling like she does. I haven't seen anyone visit her since I was here this last week. Sigh…

Dustin fixed the window; it now opens! YAY, fresh air! Thank you.

Saturday 29 April: Morning and lunch

It is a dreary rainy day. I arrive at 10:30 a.m. Mom's breathing is a bit more labored today. She is asleep with her eyes open—time for more Roxanol (morphine sulfate liquid). I held her hand, and there was no response from her. Up until now, she has been able to squeeze and hold mine. Wait a minute, we have a squeeze.

I called Pastor Todd and shared the news; he is sending out an email prayer chain within the church. Bless you, Pastor Todd.

Schedule:

- Twenty breaths per minute
- 10:30 a.m.—Roxanol
- Noon—Rolled and changed her. Thank you, Laura, Helen, and Sonya
- 2:00 p.m.—Roxanol

For the love of God, someone gave her Med Pass! WTH! After I clearly said repeatedly, *"No food or water."* Swab her mouth but no water. Then the staff looks at you as if someone killed the cat. No one reads the fucking charts! I called Christy, the manager, and left voicemails.

Scott picks me up late afternoon. His brother Cliff is in town, and we have family dinner plans. Before we leave for the evening, I ask Scott to whisper in Mom's ear. He says, *"Dean, it's okay to go to heaven and see Walt."*

27

SUNDAY
30 APRIL 2017

Saturday, 29 April

My routine for the last ten days: I would sleep until I woke up at 6:30 a.m., try to workout to keep some semblance of a normal routine, get dressed, grab a quick breakfast, and drive to Garden Terrace to sit with Mom. Today was a bit different because Scott's brother Cliff was visiting from Dallas. He was in town to visit their dad Jack and stepmother Betty. While here, he'll run in the CCVI 5K on Sunday morning. We had dinner plans for Saturday night. Today, I wasn't in a hurry to rush to be with Mom.

Over the last ten days, Mom had slept—or was the proper term unconscious? Her breathing was consistent and loud; her snoring could wake the dead. It's hard just watching your loved one lay in a bed, just sleeping, waiting for her body to give out. This is no way for a life to end. Mom had fallen and broken her hip again. This time, the location of the fracture could not be fixed. She would be confined to a wheelchair or bedridden for the rest of her life. As gut-wrenching of a decision to be made, I knew in my soul Mom would not want this for her or her family. She never wanted to be a burden to anyone. For me, it wasn't about her being a burden, it was about her quality of life. She had lost so much weight in the last six months. She went from 150 pounds to 120 pounds, maybe even less. Her skin became yellow and ashen, her face sunken, and the twinkle in her eye was gone. Those beautiful green eyes were glazed over. She had stopped or limited her food intake. She would barely take a few bites and then stop.

After speaking with the Garden Terrace doctor to discuss all the options, I called Bob to have the conversation. I am and will be eternally grateful for Bob's support and love from afar. We both agreed it was time to let Mom go. Even as I type these words, I reflect and know it was right. It still doesn't make the decision easy.

The next day, I sat with Dr. Hodges and informed him of our decision. Food and water would be stopped. Mom was to be made comfortable and morphine would be administered to assist with any pain. Mom had entered a hospice phase.

The regret I have: I should have demanded more.

I should have had them move her to a private room; instead, she stayed in her semiprivate room with her roommate who was also confined to bed.

I should have moved her away from the noisy nursing station/communal area of the unit she was in.

I should have asked for a different bed with the air mattress fluctuations to ensure no bed sores.

I should have demanded more for her.

Yet I allowed her to die in a shitty little room, in a shitty old bed with a shitty mattress.

Reflecting, having the conversation with the doctor seems like an out-of-body experience where I am floating above witnessing the conversation. I thought I heard him say, *"We call this phase the butterfly, and we will hang a butterfly outside her room so the staff will know."* In my mind, I had envisioned this amazing hospice experience where she would be doted on daily by staff in an ethereal way. This isn't a slam on the staff or the facility, but that didn't happen. It seemed too clinical for me. Every couple of hours they would stop by, check her vitals, ask if I needed anything, and then they were off to another resident.

I should have demanded more.
What would that "more" have been?

Back to Saturday, April 29. Scott dropped me off at Mom's, and I would be with her most of the day. Nurse Debbie was on staff that day. Nurse Debbie is an angel—kind, matter-of-fact, with a wicked sense of humor. She has unwavering patience with the residents and understands each of their quirks.

Over the last few days, I had Googled bodily signals that meant death was near.

Surely, key signs existed?

Google.uk seemed to always land good results. Signs to look for included increased mottling of the skin, and increased blood vein visibility in the feet, legs, and hands. Being the factfinder that I am, I tried to make sense of the process to understand it. It seems senseless now.

I would comb her hair, put Burt's Bees on her dry lips, and rub body lotion on her hands. And she would lay there snoring. On occasion, I would play a Pandora country western station or Elvis station with my iPhone next to her ear. I'm not sure if I was playing the music for her or me. When Johnny Cash, her favorite, would come on, I would sing, sing, sing.

"I fell into a burning ring of fire, I went down, down, down and the flames went higher. And it burns, burns, burns, the ring of fire, the ring of fire."

Scott picked me up late on Saturday afternoon, and we headed home to pick up Cliff to go to dinner. I was mentally and emotionally drained. I wanted Mom to elevate to another existence. My phone rang.

Debbie: *"Hi, Sonya. It's Debbie. Your Mom has changed, and I don't know if it will be tonight or tomorrow. The signs are there, she will pass soon."*
Me: *"OK, I'll be back shortly."*

I looked at Scott and with tears in my eyes said, *"I need to go back."*

We went home so I could change into comfier clothes, and grab a baseball cap, and my toothbrush—the essentials for spending a last night with Mom.

By the time I made it back, word had gotten around through the staff that Mom would be leaving us soon. Throughout the night, nurse after nurse stopped by to pay their respects and say goodbye to Dean. Each of them had a story to share, involving Mom's humor, her smile, or the kindness she had paid them. It took a village to care for these residents, and every one of them truly cared for Mom. It was graciously humbling to watch.

As I sat in the recliner, it was tough to sleep. Mom's snoring was SO deafening. At 2:00 a.m., I gave up and asked if there was a couch somewhere else so I could get a few winks of sleep. I kissed Mom and told her I loved her and that I would be back in a few hours. I left her room, strolled down the dimly lit hall into the common area, and found a sofa surrounded by quiet. I fell asleep.

I woke around 5:00 a.m. on Sunday, April 30. I collected my pillow and blanket and headed back to Mom's room. She was still snoring! I kissed her on the forehead and told her I loved her and that I was back. As the snores continued, I laughed to myself, grabbed my toothbrush, brushed my teeth, moved the recliner closer to her bed, and settled back in. Just as I grabbed the recliner to move it closer, the snoring stopped. The silence was now deafening. I popped up like a meerkat, spun around, and gazed at Mom, lying there still. Dumbfounded, I approached her bed, and grabbed her hand, still warm, no pulse. I sat at her bedside, looking at her. A flood of memories raced through my mind.

Thank you, God, for taking her. I know she is
at peace and seated next to Walter, happy and laughing.

She was gone.

I walked out of her room and asked the nurse to come in and confirm.

Nurse: *"I am sorry for your loss; your mother is gone."*

I heard the words. I had waited to hear those words uttered. All I could do was muster a *"thank you"* to the nurse.

I sat in the recliner and stared at her lifeless body. Her hair was short and straight with grey and white tones. Her skin was ghostly pale and pure with yellowish undertones. She had shrunk these last few months, these last few days. She did not even look like my Mom.

I called Scott and shared the news. He would be on his way to pick me up. The nurse called the funeral home to collect her body. I sat with Mom and took my most cherished photo—her hand in mine. I love this black and white photo, and it gives me loving respect and remembrance of the experience. I am grateful she did not die alone.

LESSON 31: Take a photo of your loved one's hand in yours. You will not regret this photo.

John Dickey, with Stanley-Dickey Funeral Home, arrived shortly after. He placed Mom in a black body bag, draped a quilt over, and laid a single red rose on top as he wheeled her down the hall. Holding hands, Scott and I followed behind. At this point in the morning, the residents began to wake, and the facility came alive with activity. I vividly remember the double doors of her unit opening onto the common area of all the wings (where I had spent the night), and seeing a couple of early risers in their wheelchairs. I thought to myself, this must be grimly weird for them to watch a dead person roll by on a Sunday morning.

Did they ask themselves,
"When would it be my turn?"

As we stepped out into the rainy Sunday morning, a heavy bittersweet weight rolled over me, and I was thankful I would no longer need to visit Garden View Terrace. The building and the staff had fulfilled their purpose in taking care of Mom.

Thank you.

We drove home in silence. There were tears. Laughs. Relief. As I climbed the steps to our bedroom, even my feet felt heavy. As I crawled into bed, the memory of the last twenty-four hours kept playing over and over in my mind. I slept the rest of the morning. I would make the obligatory phone calls later to everyone.

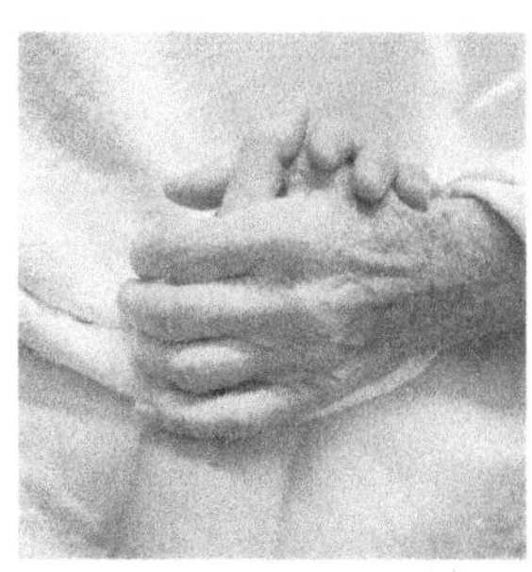

Heavy heart.
   Tears of relief.
     Sadness.
       Peace.

28

FUNERAL

MAY 2017

After my nap, I made all the obligatory calls that Sunday morning. I called her sister, her high school friends, my brother, and our friends. Everyone was supportive and offered their condolences and asked what they could do to help. It was a relief to share the end of Mom's life, even if my heart and soul were grieving.

Mom would be laid to rest on Friday, which was Cinco de Mayo, May 5, 2017. She loved a good margarita and taco. There was no need for visitation, as many of her friends had passed. A simple service was all that was needed, with a couple of caveats—no funeral flowers and a closed casket. Funeral wreaths are horrible. Three robust sunflower-filled flower arrangements were laid on top of the casket. Mom loved sunflowers the most.

All of Mom's good clothes had gone away, so I went shopping to buy her a new outfit. Isn't that a funny thing that we do? Black pants, a red blouse, and a smart black blazer were the ensemble I chose. She loved red. I attached a pin to one lapel, her favorite gold tone earrings, and the talking bear I had bought her a few years ago. I'm not sure if Hallmark still makes these bears; they were a lifesaver for a brief period. The bear had a recordable voice box where you could record your voice with a positive message. When Mom felt sad, she hugged the bear and she heard my voice. *"Mom, I love you, and I will see you soon."* That was one of my better finds to share with Mom.

The folks at Stanley Dickey did a fabulous job with Mom's makeup. Did she look like her Normal Mom self? No. Did she look good? Yes. I specifically asked for a closed casket because I did not want anyone to see her that way. I wanted them to remember her full of life, her beautiful smile, and her vibrant green eyes. Selfishly, I did not want them to see her sallow, lifeless, and shrunken form.

> *I did not want them to stand in judgment,*
> *looking over her body, and passing judgment*
> *onto me that I hadn't done more.*

It was cathartic to see so many of her church friends come to pay their respects. I am thankful that Aunt Susan, Uncle Steve, their daughter Whitney, Aunt June and Uncle David made the trip from Kentucky. As did Bob and Faith from Ohio. The granddaughters couldn't make the time, yes this made me sad and angry. Steve Smith from Nebraska even made the trip. It was truly remarkable that our family and friends came to pay their respects. Humbling, really. Mom's casket bearers included Dan McEntee, Bob Likins, Steve Smith, David Davis, Steve Wurzel, and Scott Jury. All wonderful humans who got a kick out of Mom.

Pastor Todd MacLean knew Mom and Walt. It was special to hear him share stories of her and the two of them together. They were Lucky Ducks.

Walking up to the podium in my orange dress, a flood of memories and thoughts raced through my head. I glanced down at her casket with the words *The Little Engine that Could* floating through my mind: "You can do this!" At that moment, her voice was grounding me. Sitting with Mom for the past few weeks gave me time to reflect and choose the words I wanted to share with everyone:

5 May 2017
Memorial Service for
Willa Dean Davis-Likins-Mitchell

Good afternoon,

Thank you for your presence today to celebrate the life of Dean Mitchell: mother, wife, and friend.

As the daughter of Pete and Bessie Davis, she was born into a large family consisting of three brothers and eight sisters. They didn't have much growing up, but they always had each other and counted on each other. Grandpa was a carpenter and Grandma was a homemaker. Together they passed along their values—the importance of family, kindness, religion, hard work, and love. Grandma always made sure to have dinner on the table when Grandpa returned home from work, Mom did the same. All the Davis women learned to cook, garden, take care of the household, and raise a family. Family always came first.

Mom and dad met in high school. Dad graduated and joined the army to take advantage of the GI Bill to attend college. Upon dad's return from Germany, they married and soon after, my brother was born. While dad attended college, Mom worked to support the family. It couldn't have been easy, but she did it to have a better way of life.

Upon dad's graduation, he accepted a position with International Harvester which moved them away from Kentucky and their families to start their life together in Ohio. By this time, I entered the picture and now there were four mouths to feed. Mom continued to work and discovered she was a great bookkeeper. Mom worked part-time because she wanted to be home when we returned home from school.

I always looked forward to coming home from school because Mom baked a lot! Cookies, cakes, or pies---any type of dessert was always around the house. As her mother did before, we always had family dinners. She loved cooking for others, and I am grateful for inheriting her love of food. Mom taught me how to sew, cook, and garden, and the value of hard work. She always put family first and wanted her kids to have more. Her favorite children's story was The Little Engine That Could. *She made sure we "chugga-chugged" our way to success. She witnessed the importance of education and made sure both of her children were college-educated.*

Through her love and support, she made you feel there wasn't anything you couldn't do.

She loved her family: son, daughter, granddaughters, and great-grandchildren. She saved every birthday card, newspaper clipping, and photograph ever taken or sent her way.

After our parents divorced, Mom met Walt while working together at Farris Burns. They both found a second chapter filled with laughter and love. They considered themselves Lucky Ducks and headed to Las Vegas to wed. Watching the two of them together brought joy to your heart and an instant smile. To have the second chance at love for twenty-one years is precious.

In May of 2012, all our lives changed with the diagnosis of dementia for Mom. After Walt's passing in November 2012, Mom's heart was broken, and she was lost. She missed him so much. Her illness held her back from comprehending his death. Alzheimer's is a terrible disease for which there is no cure. This last week, many of you have asked me, "What can I do?" I say, **PLEASE,** *donate to Alzheimer's research, so we can find a cure. Honor our mother by remembering her in a positive manner: happy, laughing, loving life, loving her family, and cooking up a storm in the kitchen!*

As Mom's brightness began to wind down late last week, I posted this message online that I would like to share:

Dear Mom,

Thank you for being a positive influence in my life with love, laughs, and hugs. You were such a beautiful human being, and I love you more than all the stars in the Universe. Or as you would say, "I love you gobs and gobs!" As your soul left this earth Sunday morning, I felt a presence and knew you were in a higher state of existence, free from the human form that held you back these last few years. As you join the love of your life, Walt, I know you will talk, hold hands, and share stories to last an eternity. Thank you for always believing in me and nudging me to be my best! I miss you dearly, and you are in my heart and soul forever. I am grateful to have called you my Mom.

Your loving daughter,
Sonya
#endalz

During her memorial service, we sang three of her favorite hymns: "How Great Thou Art", "Old Rugged Cross", and "Amazing Grace". After the church service, the casket bearers placed Mom into the hearse to drive her, one last time, to Pleasant Hill Cemetery to be laid to rest next to her Walter. Finally, they would be together again, for eternity.

May 5 was a sunny day with light wind. A perfect Kansas City Day! Pastor Todd said a few words graveside, and then the casket was lowered into the ground. Bob and I thanked everyone for attending the service. I went back to our Road-master station wagon and pulled out a bottle of Veuve Clicquot for a ceremonial toast/sendoff for

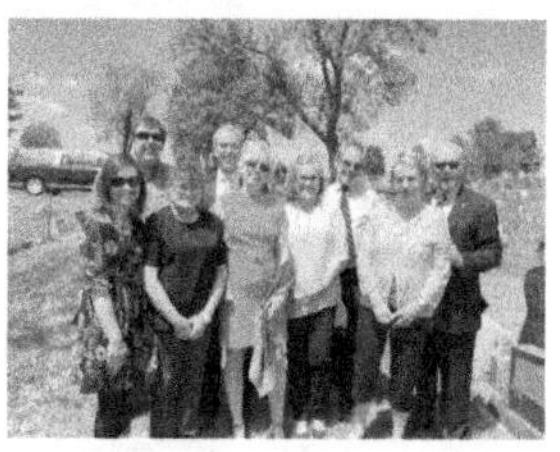

Left to right: cousin Whitney, Uncle David, Aunt June, Scott, me, Aunt Susan, Uncle Steve, Faith and Bob

Mom. Only befitting, I thought. Even Mom liked a good champagne! After the toast, everyone dispersed and went back to their respective worlds.

Funeral done: check.

29

WHAT WOULD I SAY

2023

I shared a beer with a recent connection, and she shared the story of her aging parents. Her seventy-year-old mother was capable of living on her own, and her father was currently staying in a nursing home due to a recent fall. It turns out the fall was induced by doctors who hadn't talked to each other about the ten different medications he was taking. Several of those medications would interact in a not-so-good way and lead to his instability and fall.

As I listened to her journey, the flood of memories came back—all the small incidents or stories with Mom. I listened empathetically to her. I witnessed her body language shift and her facial expression change. I watched this person, who one minute before was lit up talking about her grandchildren. A heavyweight washed over her with mixed feelings of unknown doubt and anxiety.

She asked, *"What can you tell me about your experience?"*

At that moment, I shared that I was writing a book, this book, about my journey with my Mom. I went on to tell her about how quickly stability is ripped away when you are caring for an aging parent with dementia. Thank you, Mila, for asking this question and giving me permission to write my experiences down and share them. Here are my insights:

1. Know you are doing the right thing. No matter what decision you make for your loved one, it is your decision. Have confidence in that. What works for your situation may not work for another. Do not judge yourself. Love yourself.

2. Plan for *their* future self, not *your* future self. As you know from reading this book, the first home for Mom was near her current support group, or what I thought would be a good support group. It only lasted a few months and then everyone moved on with their lives. While it will be difficult for your parent to potentially lose friends, they will quickly adapt and make new friendships wherever they live. This isn't just about friendships, it is about being brutally honest with yourself and knowing dementia only gets worse. Does the facility have the capability of giving your parent the continuum of care as they progress?

3. Don't pick the prettiest facility. Do your research on any facility. Check with the local state board and find out how the facility is rated. Do they have any issues? When you visit the facility, watch the interaction of staff with the residents. How are they interacting with the residents? My experience was that the pretty facilities were all for show and didn't care about the residents. The staff was just checking in and doing the job; they were not passionate about the residents and their care.

4. What happens when you stop a medication? In my mind, I am fully convinced Mom's second convulsion was due to the doctor stopping her trigeminal neuralgia medication cold turkey and

not weaning her off. This may seem like common sense, and I missed this. I fully believe the seizure led to Mom's quickening cognitive decline.

5. Keep their clothing simple. Socks, shirts, jeans, and whatever you can think of will go missing in a facility, especially if they do the laundry. Yes, they place name tags on all the clothing items, yet they go missing. Your loved one does not need Sunday's best. They need simple, quality clothing that lasts, is comfortable and warm, and hides food stains. In hindsight, I would have purchased three pairs of jeans, eight black or navy pullover short and long-sleeved shirts, a couple of sweatshirts, twenty pairs of black socks, and twenty pairs of underwear. I would skip the bra as she didn't need it and that was *my normal*, not hers.

6. Be vulnerably honest with yourself and the caregivers. What I mean by this is don't think of your loved one through a nostalgic lens. View them as who and what mental and/or physical state they are in, then jump ahead one year and ask yourself the question: Where will they be? Be clinical. Ask yourself: What would they want for themselves? I knew Mom did not want to be a burden to anyone. I knew she would want to be safe and as happy as she could be. Once you arrive at this decision, share it with the doctors and caregivers. Don't expect them to be miracle workers and cure dementia; that is futile. Take a more empathetic approach with caregivers. Tell them what your expectations are. I would tell every caregiver I met: *"I do not expect you to fix my Mom. I only want her to be happy and safe."*

7. Have THE conversation with your parents. Yes, we tried on several occasions to have the conversation with Mom and Walt and, of course, they resisted.

What I didn't do when trying to have the conversation: I didn't have it from an empathetic, putting-me-in-their-shoes frame of mind. I realize I was trying to impose my will and control the situation. You need to take time and gather all the questions you would want to have answers to and begin an open dialogue with your parents. Start small and be inquisitive in a loving empathetic manner.

8. Take time for YOU! This is so very, very important. Do not become a martyr. Mentally and physically, make time to care for yourself. As you are in the middle of caregiving, life, work, kids, family, dog, and career, you do not realize the mental and emotional toll caregiving weighs on you. Seriously, do not wear yourself out—it is easy to do. Walt didn't ask for help. Like any of us, he thought: "I can do this, I can take care of her." I commend his dedicated love for her, yet his own health was not helping him. Schedule time for yourself—a walk, working out, dinner with friends, a massage, retail therapy, reading a book, golf, or a vacation— whatever makes you happy. Make time to give back to yourself.

9. Be grateful and thankful to the caregivers. You will develop relationships with your parents' caregivers. Their jobs are hard. Talk about loving dedication—they show up every day and take care of your loved one. Not only are they taking care of your loved one, but they may also have up to ten other loved ones to care for. There will be times when all eleven residents will have a simultaneous meltdown. It happens. Yet your caregiver needs to remain composed and compassionate. They have tough jobs. Remember to say, "*Thank you for taking*

care of my Mom. I truly appreciate you and all you do for her." On occasion, I would take them gift cards. Learn their favorite snack, or simply acknowledge them and say, *"Thanks."*
10. There will be angst, and like me, you may learn to hate this question: *"How is your Mom doing?"*

I hated these words.

Seriously, I cringed when this question was asked. I know the person asking truly cared for me and wanted to know, but it gave me instant angst and grief. You know in the movies when the main character is catapulted through a rapid time warp of images? That was the immediate chain reaction for me. Throughout Mom's journey, my easy button default answer was, *"She is fine; nothing has changed."*

What I really wanted to say was, "She has this horrible disease, and I can't do a darn thing about it. Mom is living inside this frail human body and can't get out. Each time I see her, my heart is broken, and I feel so very helpless and I don't know if I am doing the right thing, yet I keep moving forward. I'm so sad. I feel alone and abandoned by my parent. I miss the real her."

But I didn't say those things. Why might you ask? I just don't know. I guess I felt the need to keep up this rock-solid persona—that I had my shit together. Internally, I had so much self-doubt with too many plates spinning, and they would start dropping soon. You will have these moments, and it makes you normal. Just keep chugging along and know you are doing the right thing for your situation. This is your journey with your loved one.

A fond memory growing up was a visit to TG&Y or as we called it, Toys, Guns and Yoyos.

We thought we were so clever.

There wasn't anything special about TG&Y except for their fabric department. It was my little slice of heaven. I was a fidgety child, yet I could sit in the fabric department, flipping through the pattern books from *McCalls*, *Butterwick's*, or sometimes *Vogue*. I was fascinated with the models wearing the clothing that lay within 5x7 pattern packages, just waiting to escape, to be sewn and worn. Like puzzles, I loved sewing patterns. I hated cutting out the actual pattern, but I loved cutting the fabric with the patterns. I could sit for hours flipping through those books, picking a pattern, and then strolling through all the fabrics! Touching each bolt, thinking about the pattern in my hand, and imagining that if I bought this fabric, would it work with the pattern? The fabric and the pattern had to mesh. I imagined myself in clothing design. I imagined walking into school on Monday morning in my new fancy dress, slacks, or top and beaming with pride because I made it. My girlfriend Carol was also a seamstress, and there were times we would hop off the bus and tell each other we were going home to make a new pair of pants to wear to school the next day. A sewing throwdown! It was a challenge for me to sew a pair of pants in the evening, but I did. If I got stuck or couldn't understand a pattern, Mom was there to lend a hand.

I miss that. I miss her.
I miss her laugh. I miss her hugs.

Caring Bridge—Final Posting
Thank you—25 September 2017

Dear Family and Friends,

Last Monday would have been Mom's seventy-ninth birthday. The day was bittersweet, and I took comfort in knowing she was in a better place, walking through an amazing flower garden with Walter at her side, smiling, laughing, and feeling the sun on her face.

The image posted was immediately after her passing on Sunday morning, 30 April 2017. We held hands during those last twelve days while listening to Johnny Cash streaming over Pandora. She peacefully went to sleep. I love and miss her, bunches and bunches, as she would say. I want each of you to remember her laughing and smiling.

This will be the last post for Mom's Caring Bridge website. I thank each of you for loving her and being a part of her life.

Peace,

Sonya

30

WHAT'S MY PLACE?
INSIGHTS FROM SCOTT
2023

When we are young and just starting down the road of life, we make plans on how our life will play out: education, spouse, no spouse, kids, no kids. We seem to have a grasp on how things should play out, but those plans never include the unforeseen. How could they?

For most of her professional career, my wife worked as an architect, dealing with large commercial structures. They can be a complicated beast to design and build, which means they never quite go as planned. During her career, she earned the nickname Plan B Sonya. As challenges occur, what is the best solution at the time? You must have a very strong personality to operate this way. I adopted this strategy to define my responsibility to generate a support structure. Not for my mother-in-law but for my wife.

This created a role for me. I have always been the caretaker in our relationship. It just fits the personalities of our marriage. I realized early in the diagnosis that it was not my place to take care of Dean but to take care of Sonya so she could take care of her mother. I was removed just enough that it was my role to be Sonya's caretaker. This role gave me some great clarity of the situation so I could help Sonya rationally make decisions.

Nobody really talks about the rest of the family. It is a brutal end to one's life, but it is a tremendous strain for the family that needs, and wants, to take care of their loved one. The hardest days are those when you finally recognize that your family member is no longer the same person and never will be again. The disease has robbed them of their personality and character. The stares get longer and the conversations shorter. So, what do you do?

You adapt. You come to the reality that Mom is already gone. There is nothing you can fix. No pill to make her get better. My job now was strictly to take care of my wife. To help her deal with the emotions of losing a parent, even though she would see her the next day. My job was to focus on the living.

How do you do that and not seem callus? It is a fine line and an incredibly hard place to exist, but you do it because you love your spouse. You do it because nobody else can. You do it because you can manage your own pain. Your pain will never be as deep as hers, and no one knows her as well as you do.

Our world today is very immediate. Technology has set the pace of our daily lives in overdrive. We tend to lose sight of the humanity of our existence. A journey through dementia/Alzheimer's will enlighten you quickly to what is important.

The insight of this book is to share information about a daughter's journey. Nothing is exacting about it because each person's journey dealing with family that has dementia/Alzheimer's is different. One thing is constant...

Don't lose sight of the living!

-Scott

AUTHOR'S HINDSIGHT & ACKNOWLEDGEMENTS

I believe in karma, and every step of the way in writing this book, karma was at play. I am grateful for that March afternoon cocktail in 2022 at Bar West with Mona Raglow and Robyn Stevens. The three of us decided to get together for an afternoon of experience shares, giggles, and helping each other as solopreneurs. During our conversation, we asked each other, *"What do you need help with?"* I shared my idea of writing a book. Yet I was clueless about how to write a book, and I needed help. Mona introduced me to Lisa Allen, an amazingly talented wordsmith. I reached out to Lisa, and over the following months, she became my writing rock, helping me, encouraging me, and editing my work. During our first meeting, we immediately clicked. Lisa reassured me and encouraged me to just write the first draft. Regardless of how bad it would be. Our joke, thanks to writer Anne LaMonte, *"You will have several shitty first drafts!"* I did, and they were. I wrote the first draft and gave it to Lisa for review. As they say, the rest is history. Thank you, Lisa, for your support and solid use of the red pen! You are my book-writing North Star. I am grateful for you.

I owe a great deal to the encouragement of Brooke Lewis,

an avid reader, friend, and supporter. Every time we would meet, she would ask me, *"When are you going to write your book?"* I did it, Brooke, thanks to your love and editing.

Thank you, Lynn Chalker and Pattie Donath, for reading my drafts and offering your true thoughts and edits for this book. Your wisdom and comments gave me the final piece of the puzzle to complete the book.

Thanks to Dan Viall for the introduction to Will Severns, who introduced me to Dave Stevens and the crew over at Believer's Book Services.

As I wrote at the beginning of this book, this is not a "how-to" but a "how-not-to" book. If you have stayed with me this far, I thank you for reading. I hope you picked up positive nuggets to support you in your journey so you can learn from my mistakes.

During Mom's journey, there were many friends and family who supported her and Walt along the way. Thank you to Barney and Betty Barnhart, for their friendship and mowing the yard every two weeks at the farm. Thank you, Dennis Elliot, for your continued farming support. Thank you to Juanita Porter, Verna Jean Hobbs, Marty Lykens, Bonnie Zlateff, Karen and Gary, Doris and Ralph, Wayne Heck, Elzora and Larry, Pat Ross, Michelle and Kevin, Betty and Arlen, Christie and David, Carole and Jess, Sarah and Ron, Havala and Damon, and Pastor Todd MacLean for their kindness and supportive phone calls. Thank you to Walt's mother, Terry Mitchell, for the many words of encouragement. Thank you to our many friends who supported us on this journey: David Allen, for your many phone calls filled with laughter and support; Donna and Kathy for visiting me that last week, even if there wasn't much to talk about, your act of visiting with hugs was what I needed; Steve and Randy for your love, and Aunt Susan for listening to me during the good, bad, and ugly times with Mom. I needed you, you were my connection back to happy times. Thank you to my brother Bob for his loving support from afar. I am very grateful for you and our alignment on Mom's care.

Lastly, thanks to my husband Scott for your generous support. Not only for the book support but support with Mom during her journey. I don't know how I could have meandered her journey, our journey, without your love, deflection, and support. From the bottom of my heart, thank you.

Am I scared that I am headed on the dementia train journey as well? Of course, I am! I do my best to eat healthy and exercise, something Mom did not do. I am conscious of continued learning and reading to keep my brain active. I know there is no magic pill and it is on me to do the right things. Fingers crossed—dementia is not in my future.

8 September 2017

Dear Garden Terrace Caregivers –

Today would have been my Mom's 79th Birthday. In honor of a lady who loved birthdays, please take a magnet as a token from her and the family to say, *'Thank you for loving and caring for her.'* This image was taken immediately after her departure from this world, and I wanted to remember the moment along with all the goodness she embodied and shared with others. Her laugh. Her smile. Her hugs.

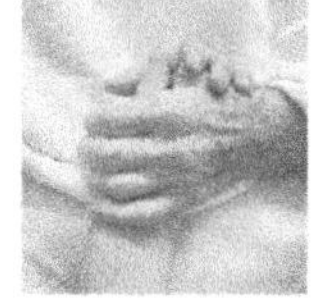

Each day you make a difference in the lives of so many! Each of you are special in so many ways!!'

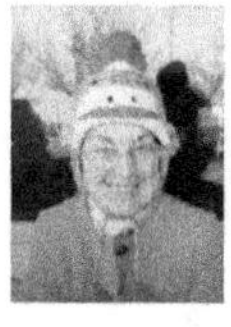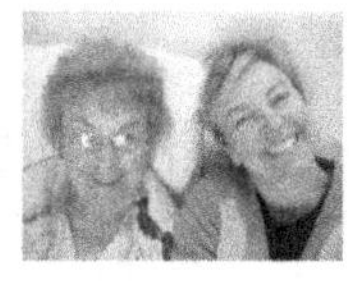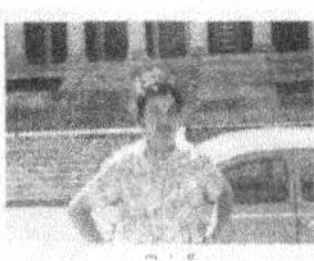

Bless you and peace be with you –
The Family of Willa Dean Mitchell
Her daughter – Sonya

"Grief, I've learned, is really just love. It's all the love you want to give but cannot. All that unspent love gathers up in the corners of your eyes, the lump in your throat, and that hollow part of your chest. Grief is love with no place to go. And as painful as grief is… all that loving is worth the pain."

—Cheryl Jernigan, 12 January 2018

NOTES

Foreword

1. www.alz.org

17. Legal, Finances, and Social Media

1. https://www.everplans.com/articles/how-to-close-online-accounts-and-services-when-someone-dies